The Insider's Guide to the New GP Contract

Opportunities and options for general practice

Edited by

Simon Fradd

Former Joint Deputy Chairman
General Practitioners Committee, BMA

and

Justin Cross

Assistant Secretary
General Practitioners Committee, BMA

RADCLIFFE PUBLISHING
Oxford ● San Francisco

Radcliffe Publishing Ltd
18 Marcham Road
Abingdon
Oxon OX14 1AA
United Kingdom

www.radcliffe-oxford.com
Electronic catalogue and worldwide online ordering.

British Library Cataloguing in Publication Data

A catalogue record for this book is available from the British Library.

ISBN 1 85775 644 4

Typeset by Advance Typesetting Ltd, Oxford
Printed and bound by TJ International Ltd, Padstow, Cornwall

Contents

About the editors and contributors

The editors

Dr Simon Fradd
GP Principal
Former Joint Deputy Chairman of the General Practitioners Committee, BMA

Justin Cross
Assistant Secretary
General Practitioners Committee, BMA

The contributors

Dr John Chisholm CBE
GP Principal
Chairman of the BMA's General Practitioners Committee

Dr Mary Church
GP Principal
Joint Chairman of Scottish GPC

Dr Andrew Dearden
GP Principal
Chairman of GPC Wales

Dr Brian Dunn
GP Principal
Chairman of Northern Ireland GPC

Dr Peter Holden
GP Principal
Member of the GPC Negotiating Team

Dr Brian Patterson
GP Principal
Chairman of BMA Northern Ireland Council

General note

'Primary Care Organisation' (PCO) is the generic UK term used to cover primary care trusts (PCTs) in England, local health boards (LHBs) in Wales, local health and social care groups (LHSCGs) in Northern Ireland, and in Scotland it is the primary care trust, unified health board or Island health board.

Chapter 1

The underlying principles of the new contract

John Chisholm

Summary

- The new General Medical Services (GMS) contract is the greatest change to how GPs work within the NHS since 1948.
- The negotiations came about following evidence of GPs' unsustainable workload and extremely low morale.
- Objectives of the new contract included giving GPs the ability to control and manage their workload, fairer pay, extra resources and improving services for patients.
- The new contract delivers benefits to practices, patients and Primary Care Organisations (PCOs).
- Features of the new contract include record levels of investment, linking resources to patients' needs, the categorisation of services, the ability to opt out of providing certain services, practice-level flexibility, improved health outcomes through an evidence-based Quality and Outcomes Framework, and a wider range of primary care services.

The new General Medical Services contract that is being fully implemented from 1 April 2004 is the greatest change achieved through the mechanism of contract to how general practitioners work within the National Health Service since the NHS was founded in 1948. The only comparable change was the contract introduced in 1966 following the publication the previous year of the Charter for the Family Doctor Service, but this change is far more radical and far-reaching. However, the 1966 contract did lead to an enormous beneficial transformation in general practice – what in retrospect seems the ushering in of a golden age. It facilitated the development of group practices, primary healthcare teams and better premises, restored morale and aided recruitment. More importantly, it facilitated better quality patient services and provided a secure foundation for nearly 25 years of sustained development in primary care. The hope is that the 2004 contract will have at least as great a positive effect.

This chapter summarises the new contract and describes its benefits for patients, GPs, practice teams and Primary Care Organisations. First, however, the negotiations should be set in context.

Background to the negotiations

The negotiation of a new contract grew out of a crisis, reflected in some of the key findings of the comprehensive National Survey of GP Opinion undertaken in September and October 2001 by ERS Market Research on behalf of the General Practitioners Committee of the British Medical Association. The survey elicited a 55.5% response rate, an extremely good rate of response for such a detailed questionnaire.

- 96% of GPs believed too much was being asked of general practice.
- 82% of GPs were experiencing excessive work-related stress.
- Whereas when they entered general practice 17% of GPs planned to retire before they were 60, that proportion had increased to 48% planning to retire before 60 at the time of the survey.
- The morale of 66% of GPs was fairly low or very low.
- The morale of 65% of GPs had declined or significantly declined over the previous five years.
- 28% of GPs were contemplating a career change outside general practice fairly seriously or very seriously.
- 46% of GPs would not recommend a career in general practice to an undergraduate or junior doctor.
- 77% of GPs believed that the GMS contract should be radically modernised.

The poor morale and dissatisfaction evinced by the survey findings had been confirmed earlier that year in the GPC's ballot of the profession, which achieved a 66% response. Eighty-six per cent of voting GP principals said they would be prepared in April 2002 to consider submitting an undated resignation from their present NHS contract if the Government failed to agree to both significant and acceptable changes to the present GMS contract and the right of the GPC to negotiate on behalf of all NHS family doctors. Ninety-two per cent of voting non-principals were prepared to indicate their support over the issue.

The findings of the National Survey provided a helpful backdrop to the negotiations, because as well as painting a vivid picture of demoralisation, they also gave many pointers to what GPs wanted to see changed. The profession's objectives included less work, the ability to say no to new work, demand management, career development, fairer resourcing, better pay, better pensions, practice-level flexibility and increased investment in general practice. It was clear that the paramount issue that needed to be addressed was what, for many GPs, was their increasingly unsustainable workload. A crucial test for the new contract, therefore, was that it had to allow GPs to control and manage their workload, and thus correct the overwhelming problem facing them.

Aims of the negotiations

From the profession's perspective, the aims of the protracted negotiations, which lasted from October 2001 to March 2004, were:

- to produce a radically different contract that gives GPs a better working life and improves services for patients
- to give GPs control over their workload
- to attract extra funding into general practice
- to pay GPs fairly for the work they do
- to improve GP recruitment and retention
- to improve GP morale.

Workload control

Many of the new features of the contract were designed to enable GPs to manage and control their workload. Those features will be described in more detail later in this book, but they include:

- linking practice resources to the needs of the practice population
- new resources when new work is taken on
- the categorisation of services
- the ability to opt out of providing certain services, including out-of-hours work
- the transfer of out-of-hours responsibility to Primary Care Organisations
- changed arrangements for assigning to practices those patients who are unable to find a practice with which to register
- demand management initiatives
- piloting the ending of GPs' role in medical certification.

Benefits for practices

The contract delivers substantial benefits for GPs, their staff and their practices. Those benefits include:

- record investment in general practice
- linking practice resources to patient needs, practice workload, staff costs, the range of services delivered and the quality and outcomes of those services
- financial gains for all practices
- a substantial pay rise for GPs
- the guarantee of additional resources for new work
- improved pension arrangements
- rewards for existing and future quality
- the right to opt out of out-of-hours responsibility and work
- increased practice-level flexibility to choose how services will be delivered
- the opportunity to make better use of the skills of healthcare professionals, to experiment with skill mix and to adopt flexible patterns of working
- a more flexible career structure with better career development opportunities for GPs and practice staff
- facilitating the possibility of portfolio careers
- the security and protection of a UK-negotiated contract.

Primary care and general practice, like the whole of the health service, have been the victims of decades of underinvestment. The new contract delivers a step change in investment in primary care and in practice infrastructure – a huge increase that at last reverses the historic underfunding of general practice. There is a 33% increase in resources for primary care over the three-year period from 2002–03 to 2005–06, with two thirds of that growth being channelled into quality improvement. This is the largest sustained investment in primary care the NHS has ever made.

One concept that is at the heart of the contract is giving practices much greater flexibility and autonomy in how they deliver services, allowing them their own choices as to how they organise the care of their patients, whilst judging them on the quality and outcomes of the care they provide.

It is hardly surprising that with such clear benefits on offer, 79.4% voted to accept the contract in the ballot on its acceptability in June 2003 – 55% of the electorate, and thus an absolute majority of GPs.

Benefits for patients

However, the contract would not be credible or supportable if it did not also deliver substantial and demonstrable benefits for patients. Those benefits include:

- allocating resources to practices according to the needs of their patients
- improved quality of care
- evidence-based indicators in the Quality and Outcomes Framework
- better health outcomes
- the Patient Services Guarantee that patients will continue to be offered at least the range of services that they currently enjoy under the Red Book contract
- consistent services across the UK
- a wider range of primary care services, delivered near where patients live
- the right to ask to see an individual doctor of their choice
- the use of patient experience questionnaires in the Quality and Outcomes Framework.

The evidence-based Quality and Outcomes Framework, which guarantees very substantial rewards to those practices delivering high quality patient care, is likely over time to lead to improvements in health outcomes and reductions in premature deaths, particularly through better chronic disease management. The Framework is unique in the world in its comprehensiveness, and has excited considerable international interest. If it succeeds in levelling up and raising standards of care, it will undoubtedly be imitated elsewhere.

The Quality Framework also provides a strong financial incentive for practices to consider their patients' experiences and views about the service they are receiving, through asking them to complete an accredited questionnaire. Practices can then consider and discuss the results of the analysis and implement appropriate improvements. Experience from practices that have already used the questionnaires has shown real benefits – the practical and symbolic benefits of actually asking patients what they think, which in turn both give positive feedback to the practice and allow appropriate change in response to suggestions made and any concerns raised.

Benefits for Primary Care Organisations

The contract negotiations took place between the GPC and the NHS Confederation, acting as the agent of the four Health Departments, which were also present at the negotiating meetings as observers. The NHS Confederation's negotiators had practical experience of the problems of primary care and general practice, experience which was undoubtedly beneficial in ensuring that the contract not only helped patients and GPs but also Primary Care Organisations and other healthcare professionals. Amongst the benefits and opportunities for PCOs are:

- to incentivise and encourage collaborative working, within the practice, between practices, across the wide primary care sector, with intermediate and secondary care, and with social care
- to expand and develop the primary care sector
- to reform emergency care through commissioning or providing an integrated system for out-of-hours care
- to improve the management of chronic disease through encouraging practice achievement in the Quality and Outcomes Framework, and thus potentially to reduce outpatient referrals and emergency admissions
- to modernise and reconfigure services, particularly through commissioning Enhanced Services, achieving resourced secondary to primary care shift and thus taking pressure off the hospital service
- to work supportively with practices to develop a wider range of practice-based Enhanced Services
- to use the opportunity to commission Local Enhanced Services as a way of meeting local healthcare needs, tackling local problems and encouraging innovative new developments in primary care
- to encourage the use of appropriate skill mix, both in practices and in PCO-provided medical services
- to encourage the improvement of practice management and practices' access to a wider range of management competencies.

The very substantial increase in resources for primary care should help to ensure the development of higher quality services and a wider range of services for the PCO's local population. Henceforward, PCOs will have four routes through which primary medical services can be provided: General Medical Services, Personal Medical Services, PCO Medical Services and Alternative Provider Medical Services. The latter route includes care commissioned from the voluntary sector or commercial providers; it remains to be seen how much that alternative to more traditional practice-based provision will be used.

The successful implementation of the new contract of course critically depends on the capacity, capability and competence of PCOs, as well as on the development and maintenance of an empathetic, supportive, collaborative relationship between the PCO, its local practices and the LMC.

Conclusion

The new General Medical Services contract places general practice on the brink of radical change – change that will improve the working lives of doctors, improve patient care and deliver the best future for general practice. It will be better for patients, the public, the NHS, GPs and other professionals in primary care. It is the right way forward.

It delivers the objectives defined by the National Survey of GP Opinion. The contract is utterly different from the Red Book contract, not least by linking resources to needs, quality and outcomes rather than to doctors and quantity. Many of the benefits the contract provides will also be available to practices with Personal Medical Services contracts; the new GMS contract has built on the best features of PMS and facilitated greater convergence between the two types of practice-based contract.

The opportunities the new contract delivers are a landmark in the development of UK general practice. They should allow general practice to regenerate, should improve GPs' professional satisfaction and self-esteem, and should produce long-overdue improvements in recruitment, retention and morale.

Chapter 2

The nature of the contract

John Chisholm

Summary

- The new GMS contract is fundamentally a UK-wide contract, although certain aspects and implementation arrangements are specific to individual countries.
- The new arrangements are principally based on a contract between PCOs and practices, which should follow the nationally agreed Standard Contract.
- The practice has the right to elect to become a Health Service Body.
- There are three types of contractor who can enter into a GMS contract with a PCO: a sole GP practitioner, a partnership including at least one GP, and certain types of company limited by shares.
- There are nationally agreed dispute resolution, appeals and contract termination procedures.
- The PCO can issue a breach or remedial notice if it believes a contractor is in default of its contractual obligations.
- The contract will be reviewed annually.
- It is the PCO's responsibility to provide or secure the provision of primary medical services, which it may do through four routes: using GMS or PMS practices, alternative providers or providing the service itself.
- Existing GMS providers have preferred provider status for some services.

The contract is largely a UK contract – a contract that is substantially similar in all four countries of the UK. The primary legislation (Acts of Parliament, and for Northern Ireland Orders in Council) and secondary legislation (Regulations, Directions and Orders) are intended to give effect to the contract documents agreed between the GPC and the NHS Confederation, on Written Consultation, which sets out the arrangements and timescale for consultation in normal circumstances. Where consultation on written documents takes place, the consultation period should normally be at least 12 weeks, other than in exceptional circumstances. In the event of failure to reach agreement, Ministers would still be able to exercise their statutory powers.

Practice-based contracts

The Red Book GMS contract was a set of statutory arrangements made by the Health Departments of the four countries between PCOs and individual GPs. The new GMS contract is a true, local, practice-based contract between the PCO and the practice. The pre-existing statutory arrangements have been replaced by a new legal basis which applies to all GMS practices. There are standard national rules and procedures, set out particularly in the Contract Regulations and the Statement of Financial Entitlements.

The national rules cover such matters as the different types of services to be provided, contractors' entitlement to resources via a variety of different funding streams, statutory requirements and how the contractual process works. At local level, the practice-based contract is individual to each practice, but derives from the Regulations and is based on the template of a Standard GMS Contract, published nationally with guidance notes on its use, that spells out to PCOs and practices which terms can be varied and which need to be varied to suit the circumstances of the practice. The practice-based contract between the PCO and the practice will need to deal with such matters as the range of services to be provided, the quality of care, and the practice's resources.

The statutory arrangements governing the old GMS contract ended on 31 March 2004. Thereafter, GPs continuing to provide GMS need to be party to a GMS contract, or – for a limited period of time – a Default Contract, based on but much less flexible than the Standard GMS Contract. The Default Contract is a contingency measure to be used in the unlikely event that PCOs and contractors fail to agree GMS contracts in time for implementation from 1 April 2004. The intention is that the Default Contract should only be used exceptionally if at all.

Even if there are outstanding unresolved matters, a practice can still sign a GMS contract while indicating to the PCO what matters have not yet been agreed; alternatively, the practice can use the more formal procedure for addressing pre-contract disputes that is set out in the Contract Regulations. One particular issue that need not delay the signing of a GMS contract is a dispute concerning the Global Sum or the Minimum Practice Income

Guarantee. The actual figures for the Global Sum or MPIG will only be known after April 2004, and can be disputed at that time.

So far as GPs on the medical list on 31 March 2004 are concerned, transitional arrangements protect their position and give them the right to become GMS contractors if they wish. If such GPs sign a default contract, they continue to have a right to a full GMS contract. The GMS Transitional and Consequential Provisions Order spells out these rights and other provisions.

Partnership agreements

Partnership agreements will need to be varied – although not totally re-written – to reflect the practice-based nature of the new GMS contract. The GPC has produced guidance for practices, giving a template or framework which practices can match against their previous agreement to see where changes are required.

Health Service Body status

A GMS contract can be treated as an NHS contract if the contractor wants. An NHS contract is an arrangement between two Health Service Bodies for the provision of goods and services. Electing to be a Health Service Body allows a contractor to enter into other NHS contracts with another Health Service Body. In an NHS contract, disputes are dealt with through the NHS dispute resolution procedures rather than the courts. This can reduce costs for both sides. The alternative is that the contract between the PCO and the practice should be a private law contract, which allows access to the courts, although contractors can still choose to use the NHS dispute procedure if they wish. Contractors can seek to vary their contract at any time, either to stop or to start being a Health Service Body. The choice of whether or not to be a Health Service Body is solely a decision for the contracting practice.

Provider conditions

A contract may only be entered into with a contractor satisfying the conditions set out in primary legislation and the Contract Regulations. Additionally, all GPs performing clinical services under the contract will have to be on the performers list and will have to satisfy the criteria concerning

If the membership of the partnership changes, there are two circumstances in which the PCO may terminate the contract:

- if the PCO considers that the change is likely to have a serious impact on the ability of the contractor or the PCO to perform its obligations under the contract
- in the event of a sudden or acrimonious split in a partnership, if the PCO is unable to determine which of the remaining partners has the right to retain the contract.

In either circumstance, the PCO should consult the LMC whenever practical, or inform the LMC when prior consultation is impractical. The PCO also needs to secure the provision of patient services. Normally, the PCO will choose to enter into short-term contracts with parties to the terminated contract who meet the provider conditions. At the end of such a temporary contract, the temporary contractors would normally be offered a permanent contract. If the PCO is contemplating refusing the holder of a temporary contract a permanent contract, the LMC should be consulted and patients should be informed.

A PCO may also terminate a contract, immediately or with notice, if the safety of the contractor's patients is at serious risk or the PCO is at risk of material financial loss.

Contractors must provide six months' notice of their withdrawal from the contract, or three months' notice in the case of a single-handed GP. The notice periods can be shortened by mutual agreement.

Remedial notices and breach notices

The PCO can issue a breach or remedial notice if it believes a contractor is in default of its contractual obligations. There are no individual terms of service for doctors linked to disciplinary procedures. If the breach is capable of remedy, the remedial notice may require remedy of the breach, identify the steps to be taken and define the period within which remedy must occur. If the breach is not capable of remedy – for example it is a one-off act – the breach notice may require the contractor not to repeat the breach. If breaches are repeated or new breaches occur, the PCO may give notice terminating the contract, after first considering the cumulative effect of the breaches and consulting the LMC, if it considers that the efficiency of patient services would otherwise be prejudiced. The PCO might also consider patients' views and whether PCO support would help prevent further breaches. When a breach or remedial notice has been issued, the PCO can also consider withholding or deducting money payable in respect of the contractual obligation that has been breached.

The contractor can challenge any notice by using the dispute resolution procedures. A PCO can terminate a contract before those procedures have run their course, to protect patient safety or to protect itself from material financial loss. However, if the dispute resolution subsequently found in the contractor's favour, the PCO could be liable for very substantial damages for depriving the contractor of its livelihood.

A PCO can also impose other sanctions on contractors, including terminating specific contractual obligations, suspending specified obligations for up to six months, and withholding or deducting monies payable under the contract.

Contract review

Each year, the contractor has to submit an annual return to the PCO and to declare that it is meeting all the statutory contractual requirements. The annual return will be nationally standardised. The annual review process is distinct from the quality review process, but both could be carried out during the same visit if the practice wishes. The review includes an assessment of the practice's workload and capacity, as well as discussion where necessary about contract variations, opt-outs, the possibility of providing Enhanced Services and any additional support the practice might require. Either the PCO or the practice can choose to involve the LMC in the review process. The review will be followed up in writing by the PCO and the practice will be given an opportunity to comment on a draft.

Contract variations

Either party can seek to vary or amend the contract. Any such variation must be agreed by both parties, with the exception of opt-outs, to which special procedures apply, and variations required by primary or secondary legislation – for example as a result of nationally negotiated Regulatory change.

Primary medical services

PCOs have a new duty to provide or secure the provision of primary medical services. This duty underpins the Patient Services Guarantee that patients will continue to be offered at least the range of services that they have received under the Red Book contract. Delivering on that guarantee is a PCO, not a practice, responsibility. PCOs must commission sufficient essential, additional and out-of-hours services to meet the needs of their population. Where contractors opt out of Additional Services or out-of-hours care, PCOs must ensure that effective alternative provision is in place.

PCOs will have four routes through which primary medical services can be provided: General Medical Services, Personal Medical Services, PCO Medical Services and Alternative Provider Medical Services (APMS). The latter route includes care commissioned from the voluntary sector, not-for-profit organisations, commercial providers, NHS Trusts, NHS Foundation Trusts and other PCOs. If GMS contractors have separate Enhanced Services contracts rather than providing Enhanced Services as part of their GMS contract, those services are also being provided under APMS arrangements. It is also legally possible to contract with practices more generally using APMS rather than GMS or PMS contracts.

Whilst the primary legislation allowing APMS encompasses contracts for all aspects of primary medical services, the power will have particular use in contracting for out-of-hours and Enhanced Services. Alternative providers will be subject to market regulation to avoid conflicts of interest.

PCO direct provision allows PCOs to employ healthcare professionals to provide primary medical services themselves. PCOs need powers to provide services as one way of addressing the contractor opt-outs allowed by the new contract, including opt-outs from Additional Services and out-of-hours responsibility, as well as allowing a means to avoid assigning patients. This new power to provide services permits the employment of practice managers where this is locally supported, and also the creation of locum banks. It also allows PCOs to provide Essential Services to patients registered with the PCO, as one way of avoiding the need to assign patients to GMS and PMS contractors with closed lists. However, it is not envisaged that PCOs will become large-scale providers of primary medical services. Any such proposal should be preceded by discussion with the Strategic Health Authority (or its equivalent) and with the Local Medical Committee.

Some common principles apply to all four routes for the delivery of primary medical services, including:

- minimum legal standards, including such matters as clinical governance, complaints handling, the arrangements for performers lists, prescribing, record-keeping and patient leaflets
- arrangements for quality, including systems comparable to the GMS Quality and Outcomes Framework and openness to external inspection by the Commission for Health Audit and Inspection (or its equivalent)
- funding via the Primary Care Organisation, from either its allocation for primary medical services or other resources available to it

- the openness of the PCO's decisions to external audit
- appropriate consultation about the provision of services and proposals for change, with the public and with the LMC.

Preferred provider status

Existing GMS providers have preferred provider status for some services. Existing GMS GPs have a right to a new GMS contract. PMS contractors have the right to transfer to a GMS contract. GMS contractors are obliged to provide Essential Services, have the right to continue those Additional Services they have been providing under the previous Red Book contract, and a right to provide the Directed Enhanced Services for access, Quality Information Preparation and childhood vaccination and immunisation.

GMS contractors do not have preferred provider status for other Enhanced Services, or for out-of-hours and Additional Services out of which other contractors have opted.

Greenfield and brownfield sites

New surgeries will be required in areas of significant population growth. For such greenfield sites, PCOs will draw up a specification for the services required, will normally invite bids from existing GMS and PMS contractors in the vicinity, and will normally only seek alternative provision if existing contractors do not wish to or cannot fulfil the specification.

Patients also need primary medical services when an existing surgery has closed or in an under-doctored area. The PCO may advertise a vacancy, invite interest from existing contractors or provide the service itself. When deciding how to provide services in such a brownfield site or in a greenfield site, the PCO is expected to consult the LMC.

Chapter 3

Patient registration

John Chisholm

Summary

- Patient registration remains at the heart of the new GMS contract.
- It is the PCO's duty to secure the provision of primary medical services for its population.
- Under the new GMS contract patients will register with a practice rather than an individual GP.
- Patients will continue to choose the practice, helped by information from the PCO and practice leaflets.
- Practices with open lists must accept a patient's application unless they have fair and reasonable grounds to refuse registration, which they may do even when their practice list is formally open.
- There is a new procedure for practices wishing to close their lists.
- There is a new procedure for PCOs seeking to assign patients to practices with closed lists.
- Practices should normally warn patients before they are removed from the practice list.
- When a patient is removed, the contractor should explain the reasons to the patient.

Patient registration

Patients register with a contractor for Essential Services. The international research evidence suggests that strong primary care systems built on patient registration produce better health outcomes and greater patient satisfaction and are more cost-effective and clinically effective than less primary care-oriented systems in other countries. Patient registration therefore remains at the heart of the new GMS contract, although patients will henceforward register with a practice rather than an individual GP.

However, patients can still ask to see a particular practitioner – either a doctor or a healthcare professional. Their regular preference should be noted in their medical record, but they can ask to see someone else on a particular occasion or for a particular condition. Whether that choice can be honoured depends on the reasonableness, appropriateness and availability of the choice.

When a patient is seeking to register with a practice, the patient's choice is helped by information from the PCO and in practice leaflets, which include details of the practice area agreed between the PCO and the practice. The requirements for such information are set out in Regulations. Amongst the new requirements for practice leaflets are that they include the full names and qualifications of all healthcare professionals performing services under the contract, the address of any practice website, the services available under the contract, the right and means of expressing a preference of practitioner, details of who has access to personal health information, action that may be taken if patients are violent or abusive, a reminder of patients' rights and responsibilities, the telephone number of NHS Direct or NHS 24, the PCO's contact details and the location of any local walk-in centre.

Open and closed lists

Contractors must declare whether their list is open or closed. If the list is open, the PCO can assign patients to the contractor. Also, the contractor must accept a patient's application to join the list unless it has fair and reasonable grounds to refuse registration. Whilst the practice must not discriminate on the grounds of the patient's medical condition, disability, age, race, gender, class, religion, sexual orientation or appearance, it can refuse patients even when its list is formally open, for example because of temporary workload pressures. Other reasons for refusal can include a history of violence, previous removal from the list or the patient residing outside the practice area. The contractor must give a written reason for any refusal, and keep a record in respect of each patient who is refused, except for applications to become a temporary resident. The PCO can request to see that record.

If a contractor's list is formally closed, new patients must not be accepted, unless they are immediate family members of patients already on the practice list. Patients can only be assigned to the practice in line with complex new procedures, one purpose of which is to deter the PCO from making such assignments. As list closures are a means of controlling workload, the PCO may decide not to offer Enhanced Services, Additional Services for the patients of other practices or Essential Services for nearby greenfield or brownfield sites to contractors with closed lists.

List closure procedure

Stage One: Informal discussion

If a contractor wants to close its list, it writes to the PCO. Normally within seven days the PCO discusses with the contractor what can be done to keep the list open, for example by shedding Enhanced Services or through locum support. Those discussions should be completed within 28 days of the notification. If the list is to remain open by agreement, the PCO confirms this in writing.

Stage Two: Formal closure notice

If agreement to keep the list open is not reached, or if both parties agree the list should close, a formal closure notice has to be submitted, and cannot be withdrawn for three months without the PCO's agreement. The notice should include the proposed period of closure, the number of patients currently registered, the proposed percentage reduction in or absolute number of patients before the list closure would be suspended, the proposed percentage increase in or absolute number of patients before such a suspension would be lifted, and any withdrawal from or amendment to the provision of any additional or Enhanced Services.

Stage Three: PCO decision

The PCO should confirm receipt of the closure notice immediately. Further discussions may then take place, prior to the PCO's decision within 14 days of receiving the notice. If the PCO approves the notice, it must confirm its decision in writing and closure starts when the contractor receives that confirmation.

Stage Four: Assessment panel determination

If the PCO rejects the closure notice, an assessment panel is convened. It is a subcommittee of a different PCO, comprising a PCO chief executive, a patient representative and an LMC representative, in each case from outside the area of the PCO that is a party to the contract. The contractor's PCO provides information to the panel, including written representations from the contractor. The panel considers the rejected closure notice on its merits, according to consistent standards, and following a visit to the contractor by at least one of the panel members. The panel must make its determination within 28 days of the PCO receiving the closure notice and notify the PCO and the contractor. If the notice is approved, the closure starts within seven days and the panel should also state the arrangements for reopening the list. If the notice is rejected, the list stays open, and the PCO should have further discussions with the contractor about enabling it to continue providing safe and effective services. Meanwhile, the contractor cannot reapply for list closure for three months.

Stage Five: Formal appeal

Either the PCO or the practice can appeal against the panel's determination, using the contract's dispute resolution procedure.

Patient assignments

The PCO is under a duty to secure the provision of primary medical services for its population. One way of providing services, particularly when many GMS practices have closed lists, is for the PCO itself to provide them. The expectation is that assignments will be minimised, but if there is no practical alternative, the PCO may still need to assign patients to contractors with closed lists. When assigning patients, the PCO needs to take a number of factors into account, including the patient's wishes and circumstances, the distance from the patient's home to different surgeries, whether contractors have open or closed lists, and whether the patient has a history of having been removed from a contractor's list, for violence or other reasons. The process of assigning patients to a contractor with a closed list has several stages.

Stage One: Informal discussion

The PCO holds discussions with the contractor, with a view to seeking informal resolution.

Stage Two: Assessment panel determination

The PCO prepares a proposal for consideration by an assessment panel constituted similarly to the panel addressing list closures. The proposal includes details of the contractors to which the PCO wishes to assign patients. The PCO notifies contractors with closed lists, other contractors which may be affected, the LMC and the Strategic Health Authority or its equivalent. The panel considers what alternative steps the PCO has considered, and the workload of contractors which may be assigned patients. The determination must be made within 28 days of the proposal's receipt, and is sent to the SHA (or its equivalent) and contractors with closed lists. The panel may set out the practices to which patients can be assigned, and the PCO is expected to continue discussions with those contractors.

Stage Three: Fast track appeal

The PCO or contractor can appeal. Appeals must be initiated within seven days of a panel's determination. Within seven days of the appeal, the parties are given the opportunity to make written representations within one or two weeks. Those representations are copied to the other parties, again for responses within one or two weeks. Oral representations may also be invited and experts consulted. The appeal should be determined within 21 days, with copies being sent to the parties.

Removals from lists

When either the PCO or contractors remove patients from practice lists, those patients must be informed of their right to receive primary medical services.

Whenever contractors remove patients from their lists, they must inform the PCO. As with refusals to register a patient, a contractor may not discriminate against an individual patient. The contractor should normally warn patients before they are removed, and record the warning and its date in writing, although this is unnecessary when removal occurs because a patient has moved outside the practice area. Sometimes warnings will be inappropriate, for example when a warning could itself result in physical or mental harm to a patient, or put at risk the safety of others. If no warning has been given, the contractor should also record why. When a patient is removed, the contractor should explain the reasons to the patient, keep a written record of the reasons and the circumstances and show that record to the PCO if requested. Sometimes it will be sufficient to state that there has been a breakdown of the doctor–patient relationship.

Sometimes, large numbers of patients will be removed for administrative reasons, such as severe workload pressure (possibly accompanied by an agreed contraction of the practice area) or the cessation of a GMS contract. In such circumstances, the PCO must write to all affected patients explaining what has happened and the options available. The PCO has a duty to ensure all patients can continue to receive primary medical services, and if they are to be secured via assignment to providers with closed lists, the formal procedure must be used.

There are a wide variety of reasons for patients being removed from a contractor's list, including:

- patient choice
- a patient moving outside the practice area
- a pupil, student or teacher leaving a school, college or university in the practice area
- a patient's address being no longer known
- a patient joining the armed forces
- a patient serving a prison sentence of more than two years' duration, for one offence or offences in aggregate
- a patient leaving the country for more than three months
- patient death
- administrative removal
- contractor request
- contractor request for immediate removal on the grounds of violence, including violence or the threat of violence or abuse leading to a fear for safety involving doctors, a partner in a partnership, a shareholder in a qualifying company, members of the practice staff, other patients or other bystanders present when the act of violence or threatening behaviour occurred.

Chapter 4

Funding

Simon Fradd

Summary of action

- Check and agree indicative and actual Global Sum or MPIG allocations.
- Agree which Additional Services the practice will opt out of providing and whether it intends to opt out of out-of-hours services.
- Agree which Enhanced Services the practice will provide and the price of these contracts.
- Agree the practice's quality aspiration.
- Look at the practice's staffing arrangements.
- Check and agree seniority payments.

Overview

The new GMS contract delivers the largest ever increase in resources for primary care over a three-year period. Funding will rise by 33% (11% per annum) between 2002–03 and 2005–06. Practices who manage the change efficiently will see a much larger increase than this in their net profits. In order to achieve this it is essential to understand the new rules and the ethos behind them.

Funding streams

The new contract removes most of the discretion PCOs had under the old system to favour one practice over another in financial terms. In future the value of most services will be nationally determined. Local Enhanced Services are the exception. If practices are offered one or more contracts for Local Enhanced Services they will have to decide whether the price is right or not.

It is important to remember that with the advent of a practice-based contract between the PCO and the contractor (the practice), payments under the new GMS contract will be practice-based and not made to individual GPs.

The Global Sum

The Global Sum covers the expenses and profits related to the delivery of Essential and Additional Services only. This is why it will only represent between half and two thirds of a practice's total income (excluding premises payments) in 2004–05 and this proportion will fall as the relative contribution of the Quality and Outcomes Framework and Enhanced Services increase.

The Global Sum payable to the practice depends on the practice list size and the relative workload and costs its patients represent as quantified by the Carr-Hill Formula. The Global Sum will be updated every quarter in line with changes in both the practice list size and changes in the attributes of its patients such as the age/sex distribution.

About eighty per cent of practices will have their future payments for Essential and Additional Services based on the Minimum Practice Income Guarantee (MPIG) and not on the Global Sum alone. This is to ensure that all practices receive as much in 2004–05 and beyond for Essential and Additional Services as they did in 2003–04. MPIG practices, of course, will also receive all the other payments that they are eligible for in just the same way as Global Sum practices do.

If a practice opts out of providing any of the Additional Services or out-of-hours services, the Global Sum or Global Sum component of the MPIG will be reduced by a nationally agreed price. The details are given in Table 5.1 of Chapter 5.

Minimum Practice Income Guarantee

Practices whose Global Sum would be less than their historic Global Sum Equivalent income under the Red Book will automatically receive the difference in the form of a Correction Factor that together with the Global Sum make up the Minimum Practice Income Guarantee (MPIG). You do not have to take any action for this to occur. This is calculated by mapping across all the payments received under the old Red Book for what in future are defined as Essential and Additional Services. The entire list can be found in Annex D of the Statement of Financial Entitlements.

> **Action point**
>
> Practices should have received indicative Global Sum and MPIG values in late January or early February 2004. If you have not already done so you should check these against your previous practice income using the mapping chart. If these do not accord with your calculations then discuss the issue with your PCO, your accountant and your LMC. Actual Global Sum and MPIG values will be available after 1 April 2004. There is the right of appeal if you cannot agree. *See* Chapter 2 which includes information on appeals.

What does GS or MPIG funding cover?

As has already been mentioned, the Global Sum and the MPIG cover 21 different Red Book payments. There are no longer item of service payments, deprivation fees and the like. They have all been rolled up into a single payment allocated to the practice on the basis of their list size and patients' profile.

Most significantly there will no longer be separate reimbursements for staff costs or employer National Insurance or superannuation contributions. The values of the final GS and the MPIG will be increased to allow for these expenses. However, this means important changes in the way you run your practice.

Staff

Under the old Red Book most practices received 70% reimbursement for their staff salaries. The employers' contributions for National Insurance and pensions were paid by the PCO. The net effect was that, for every pound you paid a member of staff, it only cost you 30 pence. In addition, this expense was tax allowable, reducing the true cost to you to 18 pence in the pound. It is not surprising that most of us have become rather inefficient in the way we employ staff.

Under the new GMS contract we shall be responsible for the entire cost of employment. In addition to every pound we pay an individual, we shall have to pay 11 pence for National Insurance and 14 pence for the employers' superannuation. Therefore, in future our staff will cost £1.25 in the pound.

This money has been added to the Global Sum and other payments. We are not suddenly going to be worse off. On the contrary, if we tighten up the way our teams work, there is an enormous potential to increase our profits.

> **Action point**
>
> It is essential to review the job that every one of us does in the practice and to revise job descriptions. Simply doing this will generate extra payments through the Quality and Outcomes Framework. More importantly, undertaking this review process will potentially increase profits by reducing the percentage of revenue spent on staff.

One of the major considerations is to ensure that everyone works to their full potential. For instance, it does not make sense to use highly paid nurses to ask a patient whether they smoke and record it in the medical record. It is also essential to do this jobs review before taking on additional staff. In many cases it will be possible to deliver the new GMS contract with your current team by simply rearranging who does what.

Enhanced Services

The two most important facts about Enhanced Services are that:

- the PCO-level minimum guaranteed expenditure floor and
- the prices of Directed and National Enhanced Services

are set nationally.

The expenditure floor

This is set for every PCO. More than this amount can be spent but not less. Local Medical Committees will have to approve that the services which are funded out of this floor meet the definition of Enhanced Services that should be funded from within the floor. This is to prevent the money guaranteed to primary care being spent on other services, for instance clinical assistant posts.

PCOs cannot use the excuse that they do not have sufficient money to commission Directed Enhanced Services. They have the legal obligation to arrange and pay for these services.

The effect of national pricing

Nor can the PCO try to put pressure on practices to agree to deliver National Enhanced Services for less than the nationally agreed price. This is the PCO in effect saying they are not going to buy these services.

Remember, any Enhanced Service your PCO fails to commission from your practice has to be done by someone else. You must give notice that you will no longer be providing the service from 1 April 2004, though there is no minimum period of notice.

The Quality and Outcomes Framework

Practices will have already entered negotiations with their PCO to agree their quality aspiration. In many cases agreement will have already been reached.

The value of each quality point is £75 in 2004–05 for an average practice with 5891 patients in England[1] with average morbidity.[2] Quality aspiration payments are worth £25 per point (of the £75 per point value) calculated in the same way. Aspiration payments will be paid in 12 equal monthly instalments from the end of April 2004.

At the end of March 2005 the level of quality achieved will be agreed with the PCO. Practices will then receive the necessary balancing payment as a lump sum for whatever level of quality points they have scored. The PCO has no discretion to vary the value of points, though they are responsible for ensuring the validity of the claim for the number of points a practice claims it has achieved.

From the 1 April 2005 practices' aspiration payments will be based on 60% of their previous year's level of achievement paid at the current year's points values, i.e. £120 per point for the average practice in 2005–06. Aspiration payments will continue to be made over 12 equal monthly instalments and the balance for quality points achieved will be paid at the beginning of the next financial year.

Other funding streams

PCO-administered funding

Seniority payments

These depend on the number of years each individual practitioner has worked in the NHS. PCOs should have already agreed your length of service

---

[1] The number varies in each of the four countries of the United Kingdom.
[2] The value increases to £120 per point in 2005–06.

with you. In general, the PCO will be able to use NHS superannuation records to verify the information. PCOs should not withhold payments pending verification of the length of service. In the case of GP locum work undertaken before it was superannuable, the doctor will have to be able to provide documentary evidence of their claim.

Using the number of years of seniority to which you are entitled, look up the chart in Chapter 13 of the Statement of Financial Entitlements to find the maximum payment to which you are entitled.

Seniority payments will be paid in proportion to your pensionable earnings. In order to do this, your superannuation contributions will be compared to the national average. If your figure is more than two thirds of the national average you will receive the full seniority amount. If it is between one third and two thirds, you will receive two thirds of the maximum seniority payment. If it is less than one third of the national average, you will not receive any seniority payment.

For 2004–05 the proportion of seniority payment that you receive will be based on the proportion you received in 2003–04 unless your practice's circumstances have changed.

In addition, if you are disadvantaged by being a low-earning practice you can appeal to your PCO for an *upwards only* adjustment to your seniority payment.

Other PCO-administered funding

This funding is available at the PCO's discretion and includes locum payments and financial support for a number of schemes such as the Flexible Careers Scheme and the Retainers' and the Returners' Schemes.

IT and premises

The funding for these will be dealt with in the relevant chapters.

Costing and monitoring the new contract

The method of determining the payments for the new GMS contract is based on the workload generated by each practice's patients and the infrastructure costs incurred in delivering services to these patients. This is obviously not static, either in terms of workload or of costs. Monitoring mechanisms have therefore been agreed.

The Technical Steering Committee is a joint group comprising officials from each of the four Departments of Health, members of the General Practitioners Committee, NHS Confederation members and Department of Health statisticians. They have been charged with doing annual workload surveys of general practice and of continuing to collect and analyse the data on expenses. Both sets of data will be used to reach agreement on the pricing of the contract from April 2006.

Chapter 5

Services available in primary care

Brian Patterson

Summary

- The new GMS contract separates services into three broad categories: Essential, Additional and Enhanced Services.
- Practices must provide Essential Services – it is responsive care that focuses on patients who are or believe themselves to be ill, terminally ill or suffering from chronic disease.
- Most practices will continue to provide those services newly cat egorised as Additional Services, including child health surveillance, contraceptive services and cervical screening.
- Practices may opt out of providing Additional Services, either temporarily or permanently.
- Enhanced Services are those services that are not Essential or Add itional Services and will often be more specialised Essential or Add itional Services provided to a higher specification. These are principally locally-commissioned services, with the PCO able to commission these services from different providers.
- There are three types of Enhanced Service:
  - *Directed*: all PCOs must commission these six services; three of them must be commissioned from practices
  - *National*: services for which national specifications and benchmark pricing exist
  - *Local*: services that are subject to local negotiation between PCOs and providers.

Essential Services

GPs clearly indicated that they were fed up with the so-called 'John Wayne' contract which compelled GPs to do all things for all people. This was one of the major drivers for change which the new GMS contract attempts to address by categorising services.

The practice must provide Essential Services. These are defined in *The National Health Service (General Medical Services Contracts) Regulations 2004*, Part 5, paragraph 15(3)[1] as follows:

> The services described in this paragraph are services required for the management of its registered patients and temporary residents who are, or believe themselves to be –
> (a) ill, with conditions from which recovery is generally expected;
> (b) terminally ill; or
> (c) suffering from chronic disease,
> delivered in the manner determined by the practice in discussion with the patient.

Part (a) is the job most patients think is the service they get from their GP. It is responsive and can be performed face to face, over the telephone or via e-mail. It involves all the usual characteristics of the consultation and arrangements which naturally flow from the event.

Obviously in cases relating to part (b) there is no prospect of recovery. This care is of a type normally possible in general practice and is not a complex palliative or terminal care package. These can be offered as an Enhanced Service if required and agreed with the PCO.

With regard to part (c), there are many chronic conditions which will impact on the provision of Essential Services but it must be emphasised that the care required under Essential Services is simply responsive and not structured chronic managed programmes of care, which are contracted differently via the Quality and Outcomes Framework or Enhanced Services.

Essential Services are not optional. No opt-outs are allowed. They apply to all registered patients and temporary residents.

Funding

Funding is provided via the Global Sum or via the Minimum Practice Income Guarantee.

[1] And in equivalent legislation in the other three countries of the UK.

Additional Services

These are services which were provided by most practices under the old GMS contract and most will wish to continue the provision under the new arrangements. Some practices, due to historic, moral, ethical or workload conflicts, may wish to opt out. This is legally possible and alternative arrangements may be made by the practice without formally opting out – or by the PCO if the practice formally opts out. The advantage of the former approach is that it may be easier to return to providing the Additional Service in the practice at a later date if circumstances change.

Funding

Additional Services are funded via the Global Sum or via the Minimum Practice Income Guarantee and deductions will be made, as indicated in the table below, where a practice opts out of one or more of the services.

Some Additional Services – Cervical Screening, Child Health Surveillance, Maternity Services and Contraceptive Services – are also rewarded for achieving high standards or complying with agreed guidelines. The reward is included in the points available in the Quality and Outcomes Framework.

Table 5.1: Deductions for Additional Services

Additional Service	Deduction for opting out: % of Global Sum
Cervical screening	1.1
Contraceptive services	2.4
Vaccinations & immunisations	2.0
Childhood immunisation & booster	1.0
Child health surveillance	0.7
Non-intra partum maternity care	2.1
Curettage, cautery & cryotherapy	0.6

Practices should:

- identify populations and develop registers where appropriate
- ensure facilities and materials are available
- ensure appropriate staff are fully aware and properly trained
- develop a programme to deliver the work

- record all interventions accurately – electronically where possible using appropriate codes[2]
- establish audit procedures in preparation for monitoring
- review the process at least annually.

Opting out

Careful consideration should be given before deciding to opt out of providing Additional Services. It may prevent a return to providing the service at a later date or it may adversely affect the ability of the practice to provide Enhanced Services. This is particularly likely if the reason for opting out is workload pressures or workforce deficiencies.

Two types of opt-out are possible.

- Temporary opt-out:
  - discuss early with PCO to try to prevent
  - usually needs to be quick
  - will last from six to twelve months – rarely longer
  - inform patients of difficulty and the alternative service provision – jointly with PCO
  - agree a plan to address the problem
  - be aware that corresponding funding will be removed
  - review progress to ensure recovery is possible
  - recommence the service or convert to a permanent opt-out
  - more than two opt-outs from providing a service within three years will mean a compulsory permanent opt-out.
- Permanent opt-out:
  - give notice of desire to permanently opt out of a service
  - PCO will attempt to arrange alternative provision as soon as possible
  - guaranteed to be relieved of responsibility after nine months
  - progress assessment at three-monthly intervals
  - after six months PCO must discuss additional measures of support for final three months
  - inform patients of alternative provision – jointly with PCO
  - cannot apply to re-provide until new arrangement ends
  - open competition for future contracts – no preference given to practice
  - monitor all payments.

---

[2] It is not necessary to enter data as Read codes. The equivalent 'label' in English can be used. See *The New GMS Contract 2003: Investing in General Practice – Supporting Documentation.*

Opting out is an important tool in allowing practices to control their workload where they have genuine workforce or workload problems. The PCO is charged with maintaining the service to patients. Standards of care must be maintained or improved.

Options for PCO in opt-out situations

- Assist the practice specifically to avoid the necessity for opt-out.
- Find an alternative practice to appropriately provide the service.
- Provide the service itself using directly employed staff.
- Arrange for an alternative provider from voluntary or private sector.

Enhanced Services

Practices have suffered severely from being required to provide services for which they have received inadequate funding and frequently no funding at all. The new GMS contract aims to allow practices to decline to do this additional work, while ensuring the patient still receives the service. Alternatively, the practice may opt to continue service provision and be assured of resources and reward. Frequently this was work transferred from secondary care but the funding failed to make the corresponding move.

Enhanced Services are optional for practices and are of three types:

1 Directed Enhanced Services
2 National Enhanced Services
3 Local Enhanced Services.

See Chapter 6 (Enhanced Services) for further details.

They will be funded by PCOs according to agreed specifications. The volume of work, the specification for the work – including quality and monitoring – and the payment for the work will all be agreed in advance and an appropriate contract signed between the practice and the PCO. Each type has specific characteristics and they will now be considered in some detail.

Directed Enhanced Services (DES)

All PCOs *must* commission these services to meet the needs of their relevant populations. They are *optional* for practices and can be refused, but it may be very difficult to become the provider at a later date.

These are nationally directed with national specifications and benchmark prices which apply throughout the UK. There are some areas of discretion but the limits of such variations are nationally determined. They must be offered to all potential providers on the same terms.

There are six types of Directed Enhanced Service:

- care and treatment of patients who have a history of violence
- childhood vaccinations and immunisations
- influenza immunisations
- minor surgery
- Quality Information Preparation (QuIP)[3]
- improved access.[4]

National Enhanced Services (NES)

These are not directed but, where the PCO and practice agree a contract, there are national specifications and benchmark pricing. Again they are *optional* for practices.

There are 12 types of National Enhanced Services:

- anti-coagulation monitoring
- enhanced care of the homeless
- intra-partum care
- fitting of intra-uterine contraceptive devices
- minor injury services
- more specialised services for multiple sclerosis patients
- more specialised sexual health services
- services to alcohol misusers
- services to drug misusers
- provision of near-patient testing
- provision of immediate care and first response care
- specialist care to patients with depression.

---

[3] Only until 2005–06 – to assist practices in preparing for the Quality and Outcomes Framework.
[4] Only until 2005–06 – in addition, this is remunerated using 50 quality points which will continue beyond 2005–06. There is a different access specification in each country.

Practices should be familiar in detail with the specification for each Enhanced Service they wish to undertake.

- Identify the population where appropriate.
- Produce a register and a strategy to keep it up to date.
- Develop a programme to deliver the work – including identifying the time and personnel involved.
- Ensure all facility and training needs are addressed.
- Put in place appropriate audit procedures in preparation for monitoring.
- Use electronic recording where possible, using appropriate coding.
- Ensure claiming process is instituted and monitor all payments.
- Discuss volumes with PCO where they may have ceilings on provision.
- Identify a process if volume is exceeded – continue to provide, defer or refer.
- Review all aspects including the contract – at least annually.

Local Enhanced Services (LES)

As the name suggests, these are Enhanced Services developed locally to address a specific local need or to pilot a new way of delivering services. They are not directed and have no national specifications or benchmark prices. The specification and pricing is determined and agreed between the practice and the PCO. They are *optional* for practices. Many practices may find it helpful to discuss proposals and contracts with their Local Medical Committee prior to agreement.

Such schemes, if successful and appropriate, may emerge as further National Enhanced Schemes in the future.

Funding

Each PCO has a guaranteed minimum floor for expenditure on Enhanced Services and this will be closely monitored to ensure practices have fair opportunities to earn and that there is no gaming by either party. The LMC has been given the role of agreeing with the PCO those services which should be counted as part of the local expenditure floor.

Practices do not have preferred-provider status for Enhanced Services (except for three of the DESs – childhood vaccinations and immunisations, improved access and the QuIP), but it is anticipated that GPs will be the most clinically effective and cost-effective providers.

Chapter 6

Enhanced Services

Andrew Dearden

Summary

- Practices are preferred providers for three Directed Enhanced Services: access, Quality Information Preparation (QuIP) and childhood immunisations and vaccinations.
- Practices are best placed to provide the minor surgery and influenza immunisation DES.
- If the PCO does not contract with a practice to provide a National Enhanced Service, that practice should give notice of its intention to withdraw from providing that service.
- Practices should use the published NES specifications to negotiate agreements with the PCO.
- Local Enhanced Services should be developed to meet local patients' needs.

Overview

Enhanced Services are:

1 Essential or Additional Services delivered to a higher specified standard, for example, extended minor surgery
2 services not provided through Essential or Additional Services. These might include more specialised services undertaken by GPs or nurses with special interests and allied health professionals and other services at the primary–secondary care interface. They may also include services addressing specific local health needs or requirements, and innovative services that are being piloted and evaluated.

PCOs must commission Directed Enhanced Services but will otherwise be free and able to commission whichever Enhanced Services they consider appropriate to meet local health needs, up to and beyond a guaranteed minimum level of expenditure for the PCO-wide area. These figures constitute a minimum level of investment aggregated to national level for each of the four countries. PCOs are responsible for developing and implementing a commissioning strategy. This should be approved by the Professional Executive Committee (or equivalent). PCOs should then consult the Local Medical Committee (or equivalent) to seek agreement on which services should be counted as Enhanced Services for the purposes of the minimum expenditure floor. This information will then be fed to the Technical Steering Committee, which is responsible for monitoring Enhanced Services expenditure on behalf of the Departments of Health, the NHS Confederation and the General Practitioners Committee.

Enhanced Services will subsume existing Local Development Schemes, the Improving Primary Care incentive scheme, services currently delivered under HSG(96)31, GPs with Special Interests (GPwSIs) and schemes to improve patient access. Existing contracts for these services will be rationalised into a single arrangement for Enhanced Services under the contract between the PCO and practice from April 2004. Each of these services must continue for at least the duration of the contract previously agreed between the PCO and the practice.

Because practices have been providing many of these services so far, it is likely that many contracts for Enhanced Services will be placed with GMS or PMS providers. However, the PCO is at liberty to contract with alternative providers, including NHS trusts (or their equivalents) or commercial providers. The PCO will also be able to provide the services itself, subject to rules around audit and fair competition.

There will be no obligation on practices to provide any Enhanced Service (notwithstanding that they have previously provided it) unless they enter into a new contract for its provision.

Directed Enhanced Services

A DES is an Enhanced Service that PCOs must commission. Funding has been made available to implement these services, where they were not already commissioned, although officially termed 'enhanced services' in 2003/4. The formal classification of these services as 'enhanced services' comes into force from 1 April 2004. The six DESs are:

- services to violent patients
- influenza immunisation

- minor surgery
- access
- childhood vaccinations and immunisations
- Quality Information Preparation (QuIP) – notes summarising.

Practices have preferred-provider status for three DESs (access, QuIP and childhood immunisations and vaccinations), i.e. practices are entitled to have these services commissioned from them by PCOs.

Services to violent patients

Each PCO area must now have a DES covering the ongoing care provided to these patients from April 2004. Paragraph 6.30 of *The New GMS Contract 2003: Investing in General Practice* clearly states that the responsibility to provide GMS to patients designated as violent will fall to PCOs, not GPs. This means that your PCO cannot allocate or assign you a patient designated as violent after April 2004.

However, if you are interested in this type of service provision you should make yourself familiar with the specification contained within the contract supporting documentation and find out about arrangements, if any, in your local area.

If there is presently no service specifically for violent patients, and you would like to be involved, you should contact your LMC and/or the PCO to enquire about progress towards a scheme and have your interest to be involved noted.

Influenza immunisation

In this DES, there will be a target to aim for but you will be paid for each and every patient immunised. There will be separate payments for the over-65s and the under-65-year-olds in high risk groups, e.g. COPD, diabetes etc.

You carry out the work as you have done in the past and claim in the same way. You need do nothing new or specific to be paid for this newly-paid-for work.

Childhood vaccinations and immunisations

This Directed Enhanced Service represents the reward element of the vaccinations and immunisations services. This money will be in addition to that to the practice under the Global Sum. It covers:

1 the immunising of children of two years and under and
2 the immunising of pre-school boosters for children aged five years and under.

This DES aims to reward the work needed in achieving these levels of immunisation. The infrastructure costs, e.g. staff costs, are in the Global Sum. Since we already have these systems in place there should not be any new work or the need for additional staff involved in this DES for the vast majority of practices.

The option to exclude patients from the target criteria was not extended to childhood immunisations. The GPC is committed to pursuing this change until patients' rights to opt out of childhood immunisations are covered by the same exclusion criteria that are in place for the quality framework.

Access

There are different access targets in each of the four countries. These are:

- England: 'by 2004, all patients will be able to see a primary care professional within 24 hours and a GP within 48 hours'
- Scotland: 'access to an appropriate member of the Primary Care Team within 48 hours'
- Wales: 'patients will be able to access an appropriate member of the primary care team within 24 hours of requesting an appointment and much sooner in an emergency'
- Northern Ireland: yet to be decided, but it would appear that it is likely to follow the Scottish model.

This DES may not be welcomed by all of us. Many feel this target is tainted by political expediency. Yet the Government has put it in the contract and is prepared to pay for GPs to achieve it. Remember, it is voluntary, there is no compulsion to be involved, only a compulsion on the PCO to provide the scheme within its area. If you feel strongly about it, you still have the choice not to be involved.

It will be paid for separately as a DES. The specification is contained within the new contract supporting documentation. While it is not part of the quality scheme, there is a bonus of 50 points (in addition to the 1000 of the Quality and Outcomes Framework) to recognise the difficulties in achieving high quality and improved access.

The method of actual payment for this DES varies from country to country. The contract documentation outlines two separate payment streams.

1   The access DES will pay you a sum/fee per patient on your nominal list. You will declare your intention to provide the level of access to your patients and then an overall payment will be worked out according to your nominal list. Of this total sum, 50% will be paid at the start of the year to help with infrastructure changes you may wish to make, or to have if you feel your practice arrangements will allow achievement of the levels already.
2   You and the PCO will monitor your progress through the year by random appointment sampling and at the end of the year if you have been able to achieve the criteria, the other 50% of the payment will be paid as a lump sum.

If you have been able to maintain your level of access for the past year, then you will also be given a further 50 points within the quality framework. This is to reward your ability to improve your quality while maintaining the access for patients. This is in addition to the payments received by the practice for access paid under the DES.

Minor surgery

Minor surgery is to be revamped under the new contract. As a DES these will have to be commissioned, although not necessarily from practices, in each PCO area.

Under the old Red Book there was a system where certain procedures were classified as 'minor surgery' and a set fee was claimed for every five procedures done. The payment was exactly the same no matter what the procedure was.

There are now three 'bands' in minor surgery. Examples of procedures which might be included in each band are:

- Band 1 (Additional Service): treatment of apparently benign dermatological conditions by curettage, cryotherapy or cauterisation (warts)
- Band 2: injections (varicose veins, joints and soft tissues e.g. tendons)
- Band 3: invasive procedures (including excisions, incisions, toe nail removals).

Band 1 will be provided by practices as an Additional Service, and thus funded through the Global Sum, and practices wishing to opt out of providing these treatments will have to follow the opt-out procedure in the new GMS contract.

Bands 2 and 3 will be provided under the new DES arrangements.

Band 2 procedures are those that can usually be done by a single person, but require additional skills. If your practice decides it wishes to provide this level of service, you should apply to your PCO. You could do this as part of your annual contract discussion or during the year if needed. Once approved, you can perform a certain agreed number of procedures each year.

Once approved you should be able to perform as many procedures as your patient population needs. These could be paid either on an item-of-service basis or as a block contract. There will need to be PCO post-payment verification so records of the number of procedures need to be kept. Just how this is organised will be agreed locally.

Band 3 is for those procedures that usually require the practitioner to have some extra training and may require an extra member of staff, e.g. a nurse. You apply for this DES in the same way. You could use the number of cutting procedures you did last year as the base line for your application. As above, if the agreed number of procedures needs to be increased, contact your PCO as soon as possible to aid their financial planning. If an increase is required in the number of procedures to meet demand, then an extension to the contracted number may be agreed. If this does not happen you should refer the patients to the appropriate secondary care provider.

The pricing of each band was set to recognise the total costs involved in providing the service as well as the experience and skills of the provider. Band 1 will be paid as an Additional Service. Bands 2 and 3 will be paid at rates greater than this to ensure costs are met and to generate income. The DES states a price of £40 for injections and £80 for cutting surgery.

It is advisable not to agree to a price below the bottom of the suggested range. If the PCO offers a fee below the bottom of the range it is suggested that you refuse to provide the service for this amount.

The specification for minor surgery service provision is contained within the new contract supporting documentation.

The minor surgery DES is a good example of a service currently provided by the majority of practices. It can maintain practice income but could be used to develop a much broader minor surgery service to patients.

Quality Information Preparation

This will be available to all practices throughout the UK in 2003–04 and 2004–05 only, although the actual arrangements may differ between the four countries. The money is to 'summarise medical records for Essential and Additional Services as part of preparations for the introduction of the quality and outcomes framework'. Simply, it is to be spent on getting your notes ready and up to the quality levels expected for the Quality and Outcomes Framework or to compensate the practice if they have already completed this work. It is obligatory for the PCO to commission this DES from practices.

National Enhanced Services

National Enhanced Services 'have national minimum specifications and benchmark pricing and includes services outwith current GMS arrangements that will contribute to the resourced shift of work from the secondary to the primary care sector. Where PCOs commission these services from general practice, they will use the specifications as the basis.'

Some PCOs will instantly see the benefits to them and the patients they serve of these Enhanced Schemes. They will see that they are indeed 'service enhancements'. Evidence from areas where LDSs have been in place for a while suggests that the schemes have led to a reduction of work in secondary care – e.g. acute admissions or outpatient appointments – in specific patient groups and represent excellent value for money.

Paragraph 2.16 of the new contract document states that 'there will be no obligation on practices to provide any Enhanced Service (notwithstanding that they have previously provided it) unless they enter into a new contract for its provision'.

This means that even if you have been providing any service now classified as an Enhanced Service (e.g. INR monitoring), whether you have been paid or not, you will be under no obligation to continue the service unless it is specified in your contract. If the PCO refuses to agree an Enhanced Service as part of your new contract, then you are contractually protected to withdraw from this Enhanced Service.

GP involvement in NESs is totally voluntary, so patterns will vary. Some GPs will not want to provide any Enhanced Services, preferring to focus on GMS provision and quality. Others may want to provide NESs that will directly benefit their own patients and then others will want to provide a more specialised service to a population larger than their practice population.

The list of NES is:

- intra-partum care
- anti-coagulant monitoring
- providing near-patient testing
- intra-uterine contraceptive device fitting
- more specialised drug misuse services
- more specialised alcohol misuse services
- more specialised sexual health services

- more specialised depression services
- more specialised services for patients with multiple sclerosis
- enhanced care of the homeless
- immediate care and first response care and
- minor injury services.

It is worth asking the following questions about NESs:

1 Are you already providing the service – e.g. INR, IUD insertion or shared drug care monitoring?
2 Is it a service that you feel you would want to provide for your patients as an extension of normal GMS – e.g. sexual health or minor injuries?
3 What changes will you have to implement in your practice to be able to deliver the NES service? If it is simple and straightforward (i.e. incurs little additional expense), then the financial benefits are obviously more immediate. But for others you may need to consider new staff or extended staff roles, increased staff time, extra training, needed equipment purchases etc. These will also need more time and effort to set up.

Local Enhanced Services

Enhanced schemes may also be developed locally in response to the needs of patients in a PCO area. These will be called Local Enhanced Services (LESs), for which the terms and conditions will be agreed locally between the PCO and the contractor, whether a GMS or PMS practice, the PCO itself or any other NHS or commercial provider, and either party could ask the LMC (or its equivalent) to support it in this process.

Chapter 7

Supply management

Brian Patterson

Summary

- One of the key aspects of the new contract is GPs' ability to opt out of clinical responsibility for out-of-hours services.
- From 1 January 2005, responsibility for out-of-hours services will rest with the PCO.
- PCOs will have the opportunity to develop an integrated, emergency care service across the PCO area that will be multidisciplinary and involve other providers.
- In-hours visiting arrangements have been clarified and alternative methods of provision outlined.
- A new contract for pharmacists is being negotiated and this will deal with the issue of pharmacists prescribing directly to the public.

Out of hours

For many years there has been a huge debate about 'splitting the contract' into in-hours working and out-of-hours working. Increases in the intensity of in-hours activity and the frequent absence of support from other members of the Primary Health Care Team out of hours prompted GPs to indicate they clearly wanted to be relieved of the 24-hour responsibility. The new GMS contract was the platform to negotiate its change.

This is a huge transition for GPs, and the public they serve, as GPs have provided 24-hour care since the advent of the National Health Service in 1948. The public has become accustomed to not seeing their own GP out of hours since many areas have moved to co-operative cover or commercial deputising services over the last decade.

Definition

The period when GPs can opt out of clinical responsibility is defined in the new GMS contract as before 8am and after 6.30pm, Monday to Friday, and all day on Saturday, Sunday and recognised bank and public holidays.[1]

Guarantee

In all but exceptional circumstances, practices will be able to opt out of responsibility from 1 January 2005. In the period 1 April 2004 to 31 December 2004 opting out is legally possible with the agreement of the PCO.

Some GPs have expressed a wish not to opt out and to continue to provide out-of-hours care for their patients. As patients will be registered with a practice, not individual GPs, it will be a decision of the practice whether they request to opt out. All providers of out-of-hours services will be required to meet national quality standards.[2]

How to opt out

Most practices will have confirmed their intentions with PCOs prior to 1 April 2004. This meets the requirement to be able to opt out on 1 January 2005. If a practice decides at a later date that they wish to opt out, the conditions to be satisfied are similar to the opt-out of Additional Services. Remember:

- out-of-hours opt-out is permanent
- no explanation is required
- PCO cannot refuse the opt-out request unless there are exceptional circumstances
- remoteness and isolation could be exceptional circumstances.

Cost

The cost of opting out is determined nationally and is 6% of the Global Sum and is not negotiable. The money being removed from the Global Sum is

---

[1] These vary from country to country within the NHS.
[2] These are outlined in 'The Carson Report' on minimum standards in the provision of out-of-hours care.

not intended to reflect the full cost of the re-provision of the service. The inevitable additional costs must be met by the PCO.

Sub-contracting

Rather than opt out, some GPs may apply to sub-contract such services to other out-of-hours providers. This involves retaining the responsibility for patients on a 24-hour basis but it preserves the right for the practice to recommence provision without difficulty. Such sub-contracting can only happen with the consent of the PCO and they will base the decision on satisfying themselves about the quality of care the patients will receive. Permission can be withdrawn at any stage if the PCO is not satisfied the quality is adequate.

Opportunity or threat?

All parties to the provision of out-of-hours care are understandably nervous about the future but the idea is to provide better, more robust and appropriate arrangements for patient care than existed under the old GMS contract.

Patients

Patients are understandably worried when they hear of GPs opting out of out-of-hours care. In reality, while many GPs will leave out-of-hours work behind them forever, many others will offer their services to the new arrangements. Some GPs may be employed by PCOs to provide only out-of-hours services. The main determinants on how many GPs participate in the future will be (a) the nature of the work and (b) the rewards.

Many GPs have become frustrated at the amount of work they have been required to do at evenings and weekends, which would normally fall within the remit of other primary care professionals. Unfortunately, GPs have been the only option in many areas. The new service will be configured in many ways but it will inevitably become multidisciplinary. The rewards will have to be commensurate with a professional person dealing with serious problems during anti-social hours. It will take several years for the new models to completely emerge but the public can be reassured that, where there is a genuine need for a GP out of hours, a GP will be available.

Practices

Practices have several concerns. First they are worried that PCOs will not provide an appropriate service out of hours and they will be left to pick up the pieces when they reopen. It has been widely accepted that there will be agreed national standards of care and this will be a safeguard for both the public and practices. It is important that this is policed vigorously and practices should highlight where national standards have not been provided for patients. Such information must be disseminated locally – via LMCs and nationally via the GPC.

Practices are worried that GPs will be blamed by patients for not being available out of hours. There is no evidence that this happens despite the widespread use of co-operatives and commercial deputising services for almost a decade.

Some GPs are afraid that the holistic care element of general practice will be affected by opting out of 24-hour responsibility. These genuine fears can be offset by ensuring effective lines of communication from the out-of-hours service and appropriate follow-up of patients to meet their ongoing needs. It must also be recognised that there are risks of underperformance by GPs performing out-of-hours work while fatigued from the increasing intensity of in-hours work. Ultimately, practices can decide whether or not they wish to opt out.

Primary Care Organisations

PCOs are challenged in being given the responsibility for the care of their populations out of hours. GPs have fulfilled this role since the NHS began and now PCOs are concerned about how this can be achieved in the time available. They are unsure of the necessary financial support, the ongoing co-operation of GPs and the reaction of other health professionals as they try to reconfigure the service. They are fully aware of the enormity of the task and that out-of-hours demand is increasing. They are aware of the national standards and the managerial and litigation risks if they get it wrong. They are not only required to find solutions to meet the needs by 1 January 2005, but they must also plan ahead to make the service successful in the long term.

The rest of the NHS

There is little doubt that the changes in GP out-of-hours arrangements will have significant impact in other areas of the NHS. Multidisciplinary working out of hours will affect nurses, social workers, mental health services, paramedics, pharmacists and dentists, to name but a few.

NHS Direct/NHS 24-type services will be developed or replaced with more appropriate structures. Similarly, A&E Departments and Walk-In Centres may see a significant change in workload in some areas. Ambulance services may come under pressure if the out-of-hours gate-keeping role changes.

It is clear that there are significant issues and the answers will only emerge with time. The key to success will be in proper planning of services, managing change efficiently, getting agreement before changes are made and securing appropriate resources.

Impossible to opt out?

In exceptional circumstances there will be practices that are unable to opt out because it is practically impossible for PCOs to relieve them of their 24-hour responsibility. These should be very rare and will be because of extreme rurality or remoteness. Mostly this will affect offshore islands, but there may be some practices in the more remote parts of the mainland included.

Such practices will agree with their PCO a support package involving financial and workforce assistance to help them in their unique situation. They will have LMC help and guidance if required.

If practices have any doubt about the PCO not trying to give them an out-of-hours opt-out, their situation can be subject to an appeal.

In-hours home visiting services

In the new GMS contract the circumstances for in-hours visiting have been clarified and alternative methods of provision are outlined. This has received little attention since the contract was published but will become increasingly relevant when the dust settles.

It is now clearly stated that the doctor decides if a visit is required based on the patient's condition. This was previously clear for out-of-hours visiting but was never clarified for in-hours activities. GPs will be required to visit if the most appropriate way to deliver the service is via a home visit. This will apply to all registered patients and temporary residents residing within the practice area. It will apply only to the services for which the practice has contracted with the PCO.

How many GPs have had their surgeries disrupted by an urgent call to a patient during scheduled and busy consultation sessions? Such genuine crises put the GP under pressure, cause patients who have made appointments to wait or reschedule and leave remaining partners struggling to help with the inevitable disruption to their patients. Sometimes, in an attempt to juggle all routine activities and the emergency, no one gets the standard of care they deserve and it is nobody's fault. Help is on the horizon.

It is not envisaged that most practices will abandon in-hours visiting. This is regarded by many as the cornerstone of UK general practice and is seen as strengthening the relationship between GPs and patients. It widens the GP's knowledge of the family situation and the social background of the patient.

Some practices due to workforce difficulties may temporarily or permanently contract with PCOs to provide for such visiting. It will be resourced by a transfer of appropriate funds from the practice to the PCO after a local agreement. LMCs would be available to help with such arrangements.

Many practices would wish to contract to indemnify their practices from the chaos where visits are required during scheduled periods of work. Again, this would be subject to agreed financial arrangements between the PCO and the practice.

PCOs will probably develop such services as an adjunct to their out-of-hours activities. They may have employed staff who would provide these services. Alternatively, a Local Enhanced Service may be offered to meet this need. Undoubtedly, this is probably not a huge priority for practices and PCOs at the outset of the contract, but will emerge as important to all parties in the short to medium term.

In parallel, the PCO and the practice may also wish to explore patient transport services to ensure patients receive the most appropriate service in the most appropriate environment. PCOs will undoubtedly be addressing this as part of their out-of-hours service configuration and it would be logical to extend it to in-hours.

Pharmacist prescribing

A new contract is being developed for pharmacists and one of the key issues which will be included is pharmacists prescribing directly to the public.

The main drivers for this role change are:

- a desire from pharmacists to extend their role
- the need for alternative strategies to allow GPs and practices to manage demand from patients and
- the political and public desire to improve access to services.

It has long been stated that 'doctors prescribe and pharmacists dispense'. However, there are dispensing doctors and now it looks as if there will be prescribing pharmacists.

GPs frequently get frustrated when patients who are exempt from prescription charges attend busy surgeries merely to get prescriptions for medicines that are available over the counter.

Various bodies have expressed concerns over pharmacist prescribing. Consumer bodies are concerned about wrong or inappropriate information being given to patients. Patients are concerned that they are being 'fobbed off' with second best and that they may fall between two stools. Professionals are concerned about the difficulty of consistent and reliable lines of communication between practices and pharmacies. Similarly, there are concerns about the protection of the patient's confidential clinical information. Indemnity of the appropriate professionals needs clarification and clear lines of accountability need to be developed.

Doctors are suspicious about the conflict of interest between professional and commercial roles of many pharmacies. Clear, unambiguous formularies must be developed to ensure the appropriateness of prescribing and to ensure that patients consistently get the same medication. Many patients, especially the elderly, get confused and frightened by getting medicines of different colours and shapes. This frequently adversely affects compliance, as witnessed by anecdotal reports from practices.

Pharmacists are suspicious that they are to be compelled to provide a service that will not be properly resourced. They have concerns over the training they will require and some are expressing concerns about work and responsibility being 'dumped' from doctors to pharmacists.

The process is still being developed, but the following is a brief outline of the possible future process:

Why?

- Pharmacist career development.
- Reducing practice workload.
- Improved access for patients.

Who?

- Not all pharmacists will prescribe – voluntary and special training.
- Dependent prescriber – initiated by an independent prescriber, e.g. GP.
- Independent prescriber – initiated by pharmacist.

What?

- Not everything – limited formulae.
- Over-the-counter preparations – for those exempt from charges.
- Drugs used in chronic disease management – asthma, diabetes, etc.
- Repeat prescriptions.
- Medicine management – changes required due to interactions, poor compliance etc.

Where?

- In pharmacy – with appropriate facilities and communication links.
- In surgery – as part of the practice team.

When?

- May take time.
- Training required.
- Premises may need to be adapting to ensure patient privacy.
- Protocols and formulae need development.
- Communication needs to be developed.
- Remuneration package to be agreed.

Barriers to multidisciplinary working are slowly being dismantled. Workload pressures and understanding of different roles and compatibility are speeding the process.

Inevitably, an extended role for pharmacists in prescribing will improve the delivery of healthcare to the public.

Chapter 8

Demand management

Simon Fradd

Summary
- £10 million for demand management in primary care.
- Distributed by a new Demand Management Board.
- Utilisation of non-doctors in clinical care.
- Closing to allocations.
- Pharmacy prescribing schemes.
- The Expert Patient Programme.
- Getting away from sick notes.
- Health education in the national curriculum.

The GPC negotiating team were charged with agreeing a new GMS contract with two essential components, an increase in profits and a reduction in workload. The former has been achieved through an increase in financial resourcing of primary care of 33% over three years. The latter will be delivered through a variety of demand management measures.

A new Demand Management Board will be set up shortly under the auspices of the NHS Modernisation Board. This new body will have a budget of £10 million for the two years 2004–05 and 2005–06. Applications will be made to this board for funding for demand management initiatives. The amount of money is minuscule when seen in the context of the total NHS budget but is a welcome change of attitude from Government.

Demand management is not a matter of saying no to the public or rationing services. It is about ensuring demand is appropriate. This is often best achieved through public education and empowerment. The end result is a better service for patients. Simple examples are the 'Keep It Or Cancel It' campaigns of the Developing Patient Partnerships charity (formerly Doctor Patient Partnership) or self-medication initiatives where the patient can immediately go to their home medicine chest rather than wait for an appointment with their doctor.

Developing Patient Partnerships (formerly Doctor Patient Partnership or DPP)

The Doctor Patient Partnership was formed in 1997 to address the increase in out-of-hours consultations. Most effort was focused on supply management, but it was recognised that demand could not continue to go on being allowed to increase unchecked. The Doctor Patient Partnership changed its name in 2003 to Developing Patient Partnerships. It is most commonly known as the DPP.

The DPP is a charity. The trustees comprise representatives of doctors, nurses and the general public. It runs 10 campaigns per year on issues relevant to primary care. Examples include 'Keep It Or Cancel It', urging patients not just to miss appointments, 'Get The Right Treatment', guiding patients as to when it is appropriate to use the pharmacist rather than the doctor, and 'Patients and the New GMS Contract', a signposting guide to out-of-hours services.

The campaigns attract enormous national and local media coverage. Materials are only distributed to practices who are either subscribing members or whose PCO subscribes. Since the abolition of Health Authorities, the number of practices covered has diminished. If you are not receiving materials, contact your PCO chief executive and ask them why they are not members. Out-of-hours provider organisations and A&E departments can also subscribe.

Practice-based contracts

Under the Red Book, partners brought about £18 000 into the practice by way of Basic Practice Allowance, Postgraduate Education Allowance, Minor Surgery Fees etc., as well as seniority payments accruing to individual medical partners over time. This was fine as long as practices could recruit partners, but for a considerable time practices have had difficulty in filling vacancies. Practices who found themselves short by one or more partners faced the double penalty of having to work harder and receive less income.

Under the new GMS contract, practice income is related to the patient list and profile. Not only does this ensure that practices are paid regardless of whether they experience difficulty recruiting partners or not, they are completely free to organise their practice skill mix.

The role of practice nurses will continue to expand to take on much of the clinical workload which traditionally has fallen on doctors. In order to free up practice nurse time and to enable them to take on this work, practices will be able to train non-qualified staff to undertake clinical duties such as reading blood pressures, ascertaining and recording smoking status and giving quit smoking advice.

Practices will need to remember that they will bear the full cost of employing practice staff under the new GMS contract and the need to utilise the full abilities of every member of the team (*see* Chapter 4).

Patient allocations

It had been hoped that we would be able to achieve the end of mandatory allocation of patients entirely. Unfortunately this has not been possible, because ever since 1948 and the NHS Act the Secretary of State for Health has been charged with the responsibility of ensuring that every member of the public has the right to register with a general medical practitioner.

However, practices will not only continue to have the right to refuse to register patients, as long as they do not discriminate on grounds of anything except violence, but in addition will have the right to apply to their PCO to close their list to allocations. This will make significant inroads into protecting practices from excessive workload by virtue of being able to restrict their list size.

The actual mechanics have been criticised for being overly bureaucratic. This is quite deliberate, because the bureaucracy all falls on the PCO not the practice. The latter only has to make the application, the PCO chief executive will be responsible for investigating what assistance can be provided to the practice, convening the adjudication panel, processing any appeal and putting forward the PCO's case, and in the final situation reporting in person to the Strategic Health Authority. Full details of the procedure are given in the guidance to the new contract.

In addition, over time PCOs that continue to allocate patients will find it difficult to recruit and retain doctors. Overall, there is now a very real incentive for PCO chief executives to try to help practices cope with their workload.

Pharmacy prescribing

The Pharmaceutical Association of Great Britain has estimated that up to 45% of GP consultations are for minor self-limiting illnesses. One of the drivers of such inappropriate demand is the fact that the majority of the public are exempt from prescription charges whereas they have to buy any medications they obtain over the counter from pharmacists. For many people there is therefore a strong financial incentive to visit the doctor. Throughout Scotland pharmacists will be able to prescribe a range of over-the-counter medications direct to the public. This will enable doctors to redirect patients who are exempt from prescription charges to the pharmacist for the care of common minor ailments. Pilot studies have shown that this is popular with the public and has a significant effect on consultation rates.

Unfortunately in England such schemes are at the discretion of the PCT. However, many are now developing this option. If GPs wish such initiatives to be developed in their locality they should request their Local Medical Committee to pursue the matter with their PCT. At the time of writing there are no such schemes in Northern Ireland.

The Expert Patient Programme

Pilots of the Expert Patient Programme were announced in the NHS Plan in 2000. The idea is that patients with chronic disease should be given generic training in self-care over a number of half-day training courses. This should result in patients who are more self-sufficient and able to deal with the everyday problems of their condition. I know of no evaluation to demonstrate a reduction in consultation rates.

Unfortunately, the programme has not been well publicised, especially to GP colleagues. As a result many misconceptions have arisen. The commonest is that far from being empowered, expert patients will become more demanding and argumentative. At the time of writing no national funding has been announced for the continuation of the scheme. If you are interested in developing it locally, discuss it with your LMC and PCO.

Sickness certification

All GPs are aware that a large number of consultations take place because the patient simply requires a medical certificate. However, the volume has never been quantified. Certainly the current system of certification is not fit for process. GPs are their patient's advocate. In general, we have no knowledge of the individual's workplace and what working flexibilities exist. Our role is not to act as the SS for the DSS.

The new contract states that 'major local pilots in large companies and the NHS will be sought to evaluate the effectiveness of in-house occupational health services as an alternative to using general practice for certification'. These pilots are now ready to run. There are a number of multinational companies and branches of NHS Plus (the occupational health arm of the NHS) who have volunteered to participate. Employees of small companies will be included in the pilots. This initiative has the support of the Trades Union Congress, the Confederation of British Industry, the Federation of Small Businesses, the Department of Health and the Department for Work and Pensions. The pilots will be evaluated by Warwick University. Everyone is keen to start as soon as possible. Unfortunately, the funding available for demand management will not be available until 1 April 2004, but we anticipate this initiative will be supported in full.

There is no doubt that it is possible to transfer the bulk of sickness certification to occupational health staff. In order to achieve this by 1 April 2006 we need the full co-operation of general practitioners. Ideas on how to deal with certification for non-attendance at court and students would be welcomed. Please contact Barbara Kneale through Developing Patient Partnerships on 020 7383 6803.

Making sense of health

This project will bring health education into the national curriculum. If the pilot is successful, all school children will have two hours of health education every week throughout their school career from September 2005. Overall the aim is to give young people a general understanding of how their body works, how to look after it, what will damage their health, an understanding of relative risk and how to make the best and most appropriate use of the NHS. The Government has made £250 000 available for the first pilot.

This is not a quick-fix option. It will not abrogate the responsibility for doctors to educate their patients. It is absolutely essential that the public receive consistent messages. However, we shall be better placed to be assertive about any misuse of the NHS.

Chapter 9

Quality and Outcomes Framework

Mary Church

Summary
- The Quality and Outcomes Framework is based on the best available evidence and is intended to improve and reward the quality of care delivered to patients. Participation is voluntary.
- There are four domains: clinical, organisational, additional services and patient experience.
- There are 1000 points available, plus an extra 50 for achieving access targets.
- Practices will receive three types of payment: preparation (in 2003–04 and 2004–05 only), aspiration and achievement.
- Practice-level prevalence will be incorporated into the payments for each of the diseases in the clinical domain.
- Exception reporting is taken into account.
- Practices will be rewarded for breadth of achievement across the framework as well as depth.
- There will be an annual visit by the PCO to discuss performance.
- The framework will be updated in the light of changes to the evidence base.

The Quality and Outcomes Framework (QOF) is a means of determining and rewarding the excellence of clinical care in general practice.

The framework is based on the best available evidence and was developed by a team of academic experts, working with the GPC and the NHS Confederation. Inevitably, as research progresses, the indicators will need to be reviewed and updated.

Over the following pages, we'll be focusing on how to prepare and use the framework as an incentive to improve your clinical care.

Understanding the framework

The main purpose of the QOF is to improve and reward the quality of care delivered to patients. At its most basic, its contents will ensure practices are delivering above the minimum statutory and mandatory requirements that are set out in the national practice-based contract.

Contents of the framework

The framework has four domains. Each domain contains a range of areas described by key indicators.

Table 9.1: Key indicators for framework domains

Clinical	Organisational	Additional Services	Patient experience
Coronary heart disease (CHD) including left ventricular dysfunction (LVD)	Records and information	Cervical screening	Patient survey
Stroke and transient ischaemic attacks (TIA)	Communicating with patients	Child health surveillance	Consultation length
Hypertension	Education and training	Maternity services	
Hypothyroidism	Medicines management	Contraceptive services	
Diabetes	Clinical and practice management		
Mental health			
Chronic obstructive pulmonary disease (COPD)			
Asthma			
Epilepsy			
Cancer			

Each indicator is divided into three different types:

- structure
- process
- outcome.

Recording and reviewing arrangements

The framework is in effect a collection of data. The best way to record and review the contents is on computer. At first glance you'd be forgiven for thinking this was an enormous task, but clinical suppliers have upgraded their systems to encompass the new structure. Payments related to the framework are intended in part to fund extra staff hours, if needed, to enter data. The consultation should not be distorted by overemphasis on data collection.

   Keeping your data up to date is important, but how exactly does it measure your performance? A quality scorecard assigns up to 1000 points for achievement against all the indicators in the QOF – the four domains above as well as payments for breadth of coverage – and 50 points for achieving improved access. How the points are distributed can be seen in the table at the end of the chapter.

First steps

There are three types of payment:

- preparation payments (in 2003–04 and 2004–05 only)
- aspiration payments
- achievement payments.

The first two are intended to assist practices in preparation and the implementation process.

Getting started

Within the QOF you can choose from the range of indicators and can control your own workload. Whether you want to work across a wide range or climb higher up the achievement ladder or both, is a practice decision. There are points, and thus payments, for both depth and breadth. In the clinical area, the disease register is vital. It is the basis for gathering the relevant data. Without it, the practice cannot achieve any further points in that clinical area.

Interim Aspiration Utility (IAU)

A useful IT tool, the IAU has been developed to help practices who are participating in the framework for the first time. It is a simple-to-complete spreadsheet which calculates the current practice achievement. The practice can then make an informed decision about how many points it thinks it will achieve by the end of the year.

The aspiration and achievement payments

The aspiration payment is vital. It contributes towards the basic infrastructure your practice requires to enable the improvement in quality it expects to achieve. You can think of your aspiration payment as a tool to allow your practice to boost its performance. In the first year, 2004–05, it is one third of the intended achievement points. Each point achieved in the QOF has a value of £75 for a practice of average list size[1] in 2004–05, rising to £120 in 2005–06. For example, if the practice expects to achieve 750 points, the aspiration payment will be £75 × 250 points in 2004–05. To assist cash flow, the payment is made in 12 monthly instalments.

The calculation for 2005–06 depends on the achievement in 2004–05. The aspiration payment will be 60% of the previous year's achievement, uprated to 2005–06 prices. For example, if the same average practice achieved its intended 750 points, it will have been paid a total of £75 × 750 points in 2004–05. This should be uprated to the new price (£120 per point) and 60% of the total will be the aspiration payment. This sum will again be delivered in 12 monthly aliquots to assist practice cash flow.

Practice prevalence

To reflect the varying disease prevalence and its associated workload between practices, a further calculation to the clinical payments is necessary

[1] The average practice list size is different in each country of the UK.

before determining the final achievement payment. The adjustment will apply to achievement payments from 2004–05 and aspiration payments from 2005–06 when the data will be available. Making use of disease prevalence enables a fairer distribution of the quality rewards because it recognises different workloads facing practices to deliver the same number of quality points. The Additional Services payments will be adjusted by the relative size of the practice's target population. There are no further adjustments to the organisational or patient experience domains.

National prevalence day is the 14 February and has been chosen not for its association with arrows and hearts, but because it is the latest day possible for data to be submitted for determining payment from April of the next financial year. If your practice does not submit its data on that day, then it will be assumed to have zero prevalence and will be treated as having the lowest prevalence of the range; a powerful incentive to co-operate with the programme.

A separate prevalence factor will be calculated for each disease area. Because there could be a radical and unjustified redistribution of resource from practices with low prevalence to those with high prevalence due to the direct relationship between workload and prevalence, given there are also workload costs that are not associated with the number of patients involved, an adjustment is made to the factor to dampen that effect. This adjusted disease prevalence factor (ADPF) is used to adjust the pounds per point only in the disease areas.

For each clinical area:
£75 × ADPF × achievement points
The relative practice list size is applied at the very end after the totalling of all the component parts of the QOF.

Clinical domain

Having created the disease registers, you can now turn your attention to estimating the intended achievement based on the information from the IAU. To discover how that achievement is turned into points, each process and outcome indicator is assessed by a percentage. This figure will reveal your points score. Each indicator has a minimum set at 25% and a maximum based on the evidence for delivering clinical effectiveness.

Organisational, additional services and patient experience domains

To discover your achievement in the organisational, additional services and patient experience domains, the process is much simpler. It is based on a simple yes/no determination. Because the full points per indicator will be awarded for achieving each one, all you need to do is add them together.

QMAS

QMAS stands for Quality Management and Analysis System. Its function is to extract and aggregate the disease register information from all clinical systems of all contractors at the same time. After this it calculates the national disease prevalence for each disease area. By referring to this, practices will be able to estimate roughly their own practice prevalence relative to everyone else. The clinical achievement will be added to the achievement data for the other domains and the QMAS will produce an achievement report that will be linked directly to the payments system. The points for the year will be assessed at 31 March.

Exception reporting

When it comes to practising medicine in real life, no matter how hard you try and no matter how logical your approach, it can be impossible to achieve perfection 100% of the time. The framework recognises this by allowing exclusion of certain categories of patients, known as exception reporting. It would be unfair to penalise financially your practice if the gold star could not be reached through no fault of your own.

Examples of exception reporting
- Patients who have been recorded as refusing to attend review who have been invited on at least three occasions.
- Patients newly diagnosed within the practice or who have been newly registered with the practice, who should have measurements made within three months and delivery of clinical standards within nine months, for example the lowering of blood pressure or cholesterol.

- Patients for whom it is not clinically appropriate, for example those who have an allergy, and other contraindications or adverse reactions, and the terminally ill.
- Where a patient has given informed dissent to treatment and this has been recorded in the records.
- Where a patient has not tolerated relevant medication.
- Patients who are on maximum tolerated doses of medication whose levels remain sub-optimal.
- Where a patient has a supervening condition that makes treatment of their condition inappropriate, for example, cholesterol reduction where the patient has liver disease.

Your practice will need to justify its level of exception reporting at the annual PCO visit if it is not broadly comparable to the overall level within your own locality.

Scoring points for breadth of quality

Within the QOF you'll find a whole collection of indicators that cover many aspects of practice activity. If you're making progress across a broad range in the clinical area, then you will be entitled to extra points paid as a holistic care payment. In addition, success across the organisational, additional services and patient experience domains will also attract extra points and be paid as a quality practice payment. This payment is determined by the third lowest score (percentage of points) you achieve in any one of the disease areas in the clinical domain for the holistic care payment and the third lowest score (percentage of points) you achieve in any one of the areas across the other three domains for the quality practice payment. The percentages achieved will be the same percentages of the points for the holistic care and quality practice payments to which the practice will be entitled.

Access

Each of the four countries of the UK has its own access targets – these are described in Chapter 6. You can also score an additional 50 points by achieving the target in your country.

The PCO visit

Chances are, that you could not manage to track your activity in the QOF without IT support. Clinical systems have been developed to enable you to track your progress. The analysis of all data using approved systems should provide accurate, reproducible and comparable results across the UK.

The information produced each year will represent your achievement in the various categories. Putting data into your computer is only half the job, analysing it is equally important.

The PCO will visit every practice, with a member of the LMC or GP sub-committee if desired, to discuss its performance with the aim of developing a relationship with the practice based on high trust. The aspiration of the practice will be accepted on this basis. Each visit is broken down into reviewing all aspects of the practice's goals. It should be an educational experience for all involved.

Where practices achieve the standards aspired to, the PCO will confirm the level of achievement funding to be given. Where the practice fails to achieve the standards aspired to, there will need to be a discussion about supporting the practice through the process for the following year.

The frequency of visits will initially be annual, but this may increase or decrease depending on individual circumstances.

Updating the framework

Over time, changes to clinical evidence, advances in healthcare and changes in regulation or legislation will result in the need to update the standards in the quality framework. An independent UK-wide expert group will oversee the process and will make recommendations to the four Health Departments, the NHS Confederation and the GPC.

Table 9.2: Distribution of points for the Quality and Outcomes Framework

	Totals
Clinical indicators	121
CHD including LVD etc.	
Stroke or transient ischaemic attack	31
Cancer	12
Hypothyroidism	8
Diabetes	99
Hypertension	105
Mental health	41
Asthma	72
COPD	45
Epilepsy	16
Clinical maximum	550
Organisational indicators	
Records and information	85
Patient communication	8
Education and training	29
Practice management	20
Medicines management	42
Organisational indicators maximum	184
Additional Services	
Cervical screening	22
Child health surveillance	6
Maternity services	6
Contraceptive services	2
Additional Services maximum	36
Patient experience	
Patient survey	70
Consultation length	30
Patient experience maximum	100
Holistic care payments	100
Quality practice payments	30
Sub-total	1000
Access bonus	50
Total	1050

Chapter 10

Information technology and the Quality and Outcomes Framework

Brian Dunn

Summary

- IT is vital to the efficiency of the Quality and Outcomes Framework.
- Computerised records will help practices for the organisational markers.
- Clinical data are best recorded and processed electronically, in particular in relation to disease registers, clinical coding, exception reporting, data capture and information management.
- Aspiration payments may be calculated electronically.
- Practices' achievement record will be calculated using the Quality Management and Analysis System (QMAS), including disease prevalence factors, which will be linked to the payments system for GPs.

The Quality and Outcomes Framework is the area where IM&T is seen as almost essential. It is probably possible to participate in the quality framework without a computer, but it would require extremely efficient paper-based information management, data retrieval and reporting systems. IM&T features in both the clinical and organisational domains.

Organisational indicators

These indicators reward GP practices for good practice in managing their information and ensuring data quality and safety. Computerised records help practices achieve many of these standards:

- entries in the patient record are legible
- medicines are clearly listed in the patient record
- drug allergies and intolerances are recorded
- there are clearly-defined arrangements for computer data backup and storage
- details of prescribed medicines are available at each surgery consultation.

Clinical indicators

Practices that wish to maximise their incomes and patient care under the quality clinical indicators will find life much easier if they possess and extensively use their computers. It is now probably more important that clinical data are recorded electronically than on the paper record. All the main clinical system suppliers are responding to the requirements practices will have under the new contract and data capture will be aided to ensure ease and consistency of recording. The main requirements practices have in the early months of the contract are as follows.

- *Disease registers*: Practices cannot gain any clinical points in any disease category unless they have a register for that disease. Populating the disease registers will be aided by the system suppliers as they modify their software to comply with the requirements for the contract, but it is essential that practices ensure their registers are accurate and up to date. Practices that expend time now in forming and updating disease registers will be in a better position to achieve higher points totals in March 2005.
- *Clinical coding*: Data extraction for quality achievements will in most cases be electronic. It is essential that practices code the measurable outcomes in the correct fashion. Many individuals and organisations are attempting to produce formularies and search engines to help practices at present. Practices should not be enticed into wasting time with unofficial products. The NHS Information Authority has released the preferred Read codes to the system suppliers and these are available on the Web at www.nhsia. nhs.uk/terms/pages/default.asp. However, practice systems will allow GPs and staff to enter diagnoses in English or by template with mapping to the appropriate Read code.

- *Exception reporting*: It is essential that Read codes for the exception reporting aspect of the Quality and Outcomes Framework are satisfactory. Exception reporting is a new concept to GPs and the system suppliers and codes for contraindications, on maximal therapy etc. must give accurate results with the data extraction tools.
- *Data capture*: Practices should have in place systems for capturing data from outwith the practice. Many discharge and outpatient letters from acute providers contain codeable data and it is not sufficient to record the diagnosis/procedure. Blood pressures, HbA1Cs, results of CT scans, echocardiograms, U&Es, thyroid function tests, lung function tests, exercise ECGs etc. should be identified from the clinical letter and recorded on the practice system as a Read code. Practices should have such systems in place and all staff responsible for scanning/filing letters should be aware of the policy and have time to enter the data.
- *Information management*: The latest software is of little use if practices do not have a robust information management system. All members of the primary care team (including attached nurses and health visitors) should have access to computer terminals and have had training to enable data entry on the practice computer system. Practices must ensure that all data are recorded on the practice computer system – before or instead of entering on paper records.
- *Reluctant computer users*: Practices can no longer afford the GP or nurse who cannot or will not enter data on the computer. Adequate training and time should be given to all staff to enable this. Data recording may well be covered in practice partnership agreements and in cases where a GP or member of staff cannot record data adequately for GMS purposes, the practice may have to make alternative arrangements for the data entry while the GP continues to perform the clinical duties.

Calculation of aspiration points

In year one, quality aspiration points will be calculated using an Excel spreadsheet called the Interim Aspiration Utility. This spreadsheet will not take data from the practice computer system, but practices should have some data to justify their aspiration, as it must be realistic. From 2005–06 onwards, aspiration points will be agreed with the PCO based on the previous year's achievement level and any changes that may have occurred within the practice that may either increase or decrease the level of aspiration.

Calculation of achievement

It is intended that practice achievement will be calculated using a tool that is being developed called the Quality and Outcomes Management and Analysis System (QMAS). This will also allow national and practice prevalence of disease to be calculated.

It is intended that QMAS will work with RFA[1] practice systems and extract clinical data automatically from the clinical system while the organisational, patient experience and additional services markers will be entered manually by the practice via a web-based interface. It is hoped that QMAS will be operational by August 2004. QMAS will enable practices to:

- assess their current quality achievement points, estimated relative prevalence and current achievement payment whenever they wish
- compare their current position with the average achievement in the PCT, the SHA and nationally. Such comparisons would not involve disclosure of information that identifies other contractors. This facility will be available later after the main system has gone live
- check that the data they are providing are correct and complete.

Data will flow from QMAS to the payment system for GP payments. Prevalence will be calculated in February and payment to practices using their actual achievement points adjusted for list size and practice disease prevalence against national prevalence will be paid to practices as a lump sum in April of the next financial year.

Operation of QMAS

The data flows are illustrated in Figure 10.1.[2]

There will also be a data flow from QMAS to PCOs. These data will be anonymised to allow PCOs to track the global points total in their area for financial planning. It is important for PCOs to know if practices are over-performing in quality well before the end of the financial year, as they will have to pay GPs. Equally, it is important if there is significant under-performance, as GMS monies may have to be allocated to other areas such as Enhanced Services. PCOs will also be able to compare achievement levels and disease prevalence against other PCOs and this may help them target

---

[1] *See* Appendix.
[2] Source: *Delivering Investment in General Practice*, Department of Health.

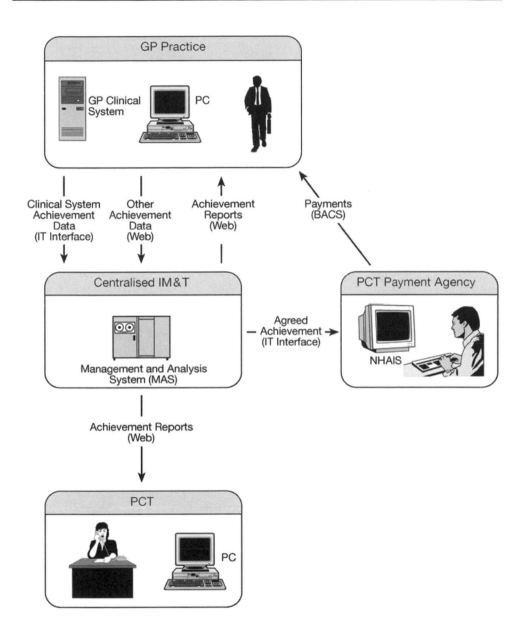

Figure 10.1: Data flows.

resources at practices or learn from practice support given by PCOs performing at a higher level.

This system will be procured by the National Programme for IT (NPfIT) and it can be seen to fit in with Government Integrated Care Records Service (ICRS) policy. It is not, however, intended that GPs will be performance-managed using this system. PCOs have been instructed in the use of the system and contractor identifiable information will only be made available to the PCO at its request if there is a suspicion of serious fraud.

Chapter 11

Information technology

Brian Dunn

Summary
- The contract promises in excess of £100 million investment in Information Technology in England in 2004–05 and 2005–06, with equivalent sums for Scotland, Wales and Northern Ireland.
- PCOs will in future own the IT systems in practices and will bear the total capital and maintenance costs.
- GPs are guaranteed a choice from a number of accredited systems.
- PCOs will be responsible for training GPs and other primary care staff in the use of their IT systems.

Funding for IM&T in the new GMS contract

IM&T takes up only a few pages of the contract documentation. The contract, however, promises unparalleled investment in general practice infrastructure, including information technology. The supporting documentation to the contract promises in excess of £100 million investment in England in 2004–05 and 2005–06, with equivalent sums for Scotland, Wales and Northern Ireland. The three Celtic countries appear to be happiest about this element of the contract, as their devolved administrations have made the promised amounts available in 2003–04 for minor upgrades and maintenance. The English funding has become rather more difficult to identify because the responsibility for funding lies with the National Programme for IT, which is NHS-wide.

This is an important area for the General Practitioners Committee and Local Medical Committees, who must monitor practices to ensure they are adequately equipped with IT systems that are fit for purpose to enable GPs and their staff to deliver the benefits of the contract to their practices and patients.

Primary care IM&T: the future

The new GMS contract heralds a major change in the future development of IM&T. Instead of the piecemeal development seen up until now, the contract document promises 'integration at a community level' and 'national IM&T programmes'. The intention is for GPs to receive an information technology service rather than purchasing the hardware and software. The concept of GPs receiving reimbursement for the system of their choice regardless of other local priorities has gone. As systems are replaced, PCOs will in future own the IT systems in practices and will bear the total capital and maintenance costs. GPs are guaranteed a choice from a number of accredited systems, and issues such as confidentiality, liability and training are addressed.

For an historical perspective and an outline of the vision for IT in general practice as part of the wider NHS context, *see* the Appendix on pp. 161–164.

Ownership of IT systems

Traditionally, practices have owned their IT systems. This applied to fund-holding systems where the practice received 100% reimbursement and ownership of the systems remained with the GP practice. GPs have always zealously guarded the information contained in their electronic and paper patient records. This was to preserve confidentiality of clinical information – much of which was imparted to the GP on the implicit understanding by the patient that it would not be divulged inappropriately to a third party. GPs have also resisted PCO access to data as they fear performance management by PCOs.

Under the terms of the new GMS contract, PCOs will own the practice IT systems. Initially, practice systems will remain in the ownership of practices that have purchased them. However, as systems become dated and hardware and software are replaced, the PCO will own a greater proportion of the practice IT system until eventually the PCO will own the totality of the system. This leaves practices with some dilemmas and decisions to make. Issues to be considered include the following.

- *Confidentiality*: The GP's relationship with their patients is based on trust. Patients do not expect GPs to divulge information imparted confidentially in the course of a consultation to others except when it is to be used for the further clinical care of the patient or with the informed consent of the patient. It is important that this relationship is maintained under the new contract.

- *Choice of system*: It is envisaged that most GP practices will continue with their current system supplier. Changing systems is an enormous upheaval for practices – GPs and clerical staff and up to 30% of clinical data may be lost transferring data between systems. The contract guarantees GPs a choice of system with a right to change suppliers every three years. It is unlikely that choice will be unlimited but it is anticipated that practices will have a choice of three to four systems that are consistent with the PCO Local Development Plan. Practices will be required to support bids for new hardware or change of supplier with a business case and changing system supplier may be permitted in less than three years if the practice can demonstrate failure of the software to meet contractual demands or where the maintenance does not meet the standards set out in the SLA. One important role for LMCs and the GPC will be to ensure that practices have genuine choice of systems and that Local Service Providers (LSPs) do not force practices to change computer systems.
- *Maintenance*: Most practices presently have maintenance contracts with their system suppliers. These cover either software or software and hardware combined. The contracts have quality standards and defined time limits for fixing problems according to the impact the problem is having on the running of the practice. It is essential that the Service Level Agreements (SLA) between the practice, supplier and PCO offer at least as good service. The contract guarantees practices 100% reimbursement of maintenance of existing systems.
- *Liability*: As GPs will no longer own their IT systems, they will input patient data into a computer owned by the PCO. NHS organisations do not insure hardware. Practices must ensure that SLAs cover the replacement of damaged or stolen systems and the restoration of data in a timely manner. The issue of liability in the case of patient harm due to the unavailability of electronic data should be addressed in the agreement the practice has with the PCO.
- *Other software*: Many practices use their clinical workstations to install other software to help run their practices – word processing, spreadsheets, accounts and other clinical and non-clinical applications. PCOs may well limit the applications they will allow practices to install on their computers and practices may need to (or prefer to) buy stand-alone computers for purposes such as practice accounts and other non-clinical data so they will not be accessible to the PCO.
- *Training*: PCOs will be responsible for training GPs and other primary care staff in the use of their IT systems. It is essential that the substantial

investment in IM&T delivered by the new GMS contract is supported by adequate training and the GPC is working with the devolved administrations to ensure resources are allocated to allow practices access to training.

- *GP-to-GP transfer of records*: The GP-to-GP project was in the process of development by the Health Department in England during negotiations on the new contract. The GPC argued and the NHS Confederation and the Department accepted its case, that this should be made a UK-wide project to aid practices and to facilitate the maintenance of data quality. New patients have a weighting in the Carr-Hill formula because of the extra work in recording the health, immunisation and therapy record of a new patient. This work obviously takes place in the first year of their registration and areas (such as inner cities) that have high list turnover have an inordinate amount of work to keep their records up to date. Electronic transfer of data from GP practice to new GP practice will alleviate much of this work, although there are problems with the new practice having to:
  - verify the data quality
  - consider how to correct inaccurate data without altering historic records
  - mark data recorded by other practices, as there may be differences in how different practices code and treat various diseases
  - decide how to integrate the historic data within their own records.

Chapter 12

Practice premises

Peter Holden

Summary

- Modern primary care requires more than the simple GP surgery – proposals for one-stop developments (incorporating pharmacy, dentistry, physiotherapy and other health and social care service providers) are more likely to receive funding approval than simpler models of premises provision.
- The underlying philosophy behind NHS rental of GP premises developments is to achieve a state where practices operate from quality premises fit for purpose of adequate size, specification and flexibility to support delivery of modern high quality care.
- PCOs are required to consider applications for financial assistance towards premises development and improvement where a practice wishes to build, purchase, develop or improve premises for the delivery of primary medical services.
- Practices contemplating premises development must discuss matters with their LMC and PCO before incurring professional fees in preparing a bid for premises monies.
- Premises is the one area where it is essential to take specialist professional advice.
- Improvement grants ranging in value from 33% to 66% of the project costs are available subject to PCO discretion and budgetary constraints.
- Funds for premises development are held by a lead PCT on a Strategic Health Authority-wide basis.
- New flexibilities in premises funding have been introduced.
- Minimum standards are now set out in Directions for surgery premises.
- Notional rent payments continue and cost rent payments (renamed as borrowing costs reimbursements) remain.
- Payments made under the premises Directions require the initiative to come from the practice to claim them.

Introduction

Even in the current uncertain property climate, surgery premises investment has proved to deliver a good return in the long run. It is for this reason that third party developers still have a healthy interest in this specialist investment market. The definitive text governing practice premises under the new GMS contract is *The National Health Service (General Medical Services – Premises Costs) (England) Directions 2004* and the parallel Directions in Wales, Northern Ireland and Scotland. If you are contemplating practice premises development there is no alternative but to get your head around these regulations. Anyone who has developed practice premises in the past knows how complicated are the relevant rules and regulations. Many GPs are content to leave these technicalities to an enthusiastic partner as project overseer.

The good news in the new GMS contract is that, for those practices which are not currently involved in building projects or contemplating such projects, it is very much business as usual, with borrowing costs reimbursement (formerly cost rent) and notional rent payments continuing without change. Such monies form part of the guaranteed baseline funding of PCOs (paragraph 5.40 of *The New GMS Contract 2003: Investing in General Practice*) and will be uplifted each year for property cost inflation as advised by the Valuation Office Agency. It is noticeable that the term 'cost rent' is disappearing although the concept and practice of reimbursing practice premises borrowing costs in full remains. It is now possible to receive both notional rent and cost rent on premises where an extension has been constructed and yet the extended building is rated with a current market rent of less than the cost rent. It is also possible for notional rent to be paid upon leasehold premises where the GP tenant has carried out approved improvements that are not covered by the rent reimbursement. Payments made under the premises Directions require the initiative to come from the practice to claim them.

Purchase or lease?

Premises is one area of the new GMS contract where it is essential to take *specialist* professional advice. GP surgery premises are now specialist, purpose-built premises rather than converted domestic buildings. Such developments do not have the potential for easy conversion to other uses and, particularly in the design and valuation aspects of such projects, it is essential that specialist architects, surveyors and valuers are commissioned to ensure maximum return on the commercial investment that you are contemplating.

Nowadays these projects are not purely exercises in obtaining good premises fit for purpose – but the foundation for a successful practice with financial viability guaranteed through the erstwhile one-way bet on property values. It is now essential to ensure that good design produces a pleasing result that is professionally efficient to operate and economical with maintenance costs. Financial viability must also be built in by careful selection of funding mechanisms for the project. Employing the local architect or domestic valuer for your project is likely to prove a false economy in the long run unless they happen to be specialists in GP premises.

Although the profession is moving towards portfolio career structures, a sizeable number of doctors are still prepared to make a long-term commitment to the area and the practice which they join. The benefits of tax-efficient investment opportunities in surgery property still hold true for the long term. If this were untrue, then third party developers (TPDs) would not be taking such an interest in the sector, and the financial institutions would not offer such preferential lending terms on GP surgery projects.

Modern primary care requires a broader vision of surgery premises than the simple GP and nurse consulting room/treatment room/office reception/waiting room model of premises extant until recently. The trend is more towards one-stop single location healthcare, incorporating pharmacy, dentistry, physiotherapy and other health and social care service providers. Such development proposals accord with Government policy and are more likely to receive funding approval than older models of premises provision. Space for other contractors can either be provided on a lease basis with the GPs as landlords or GPs can become involved in joint funding arrangements. Where GPs choose to be owner-occupiers of premises they will continue to need to exercise the 'prudent businessman' approach to a project that will have to stack up in financial terms.

Alternatively a third party developer (TPD) might develop a project on a Private Finance Initiative (PFI) lease-type arrangement, in which case the GP will have no investment in the property but will almost certainly have long-term contractual obligations in respect of the property as the leaseholder. For a fuller exposition on premises and funding structures the reader is directed to *The Future of GP Practice Premises: guidance for GPs* – available at www.bma. org.uk which is regularly updated.

The underlying philosophy behind GP premises developments and their rental by the NHS is to achieve a state where practices operate from quality premises fit for purpose of adequate size, specification and flexibility to support delivery of modern high quality care.

Many GPs were frustrated by the limitations of the old Red Book provisions applicable to premises which failed to reflect modern patterns of provision of primary care and were predicated upon the number of doctor partners. Except in Health Action Zones, the former Red Book provisions only dealt with one half of the premises development problem – the funding of new or improved premises. The Red Book did nothing to address the fact that viability of a new premises project was frequently critically dependent on the ability to dispose of current surgery premises without financial loss to the GP.

Premises development proposals

PCOs are required formally to consider all applications for financial assist-ance towards premises development and improvement where a practice wishes to build, purchase, develop or improve premises for the delivery of primary medical services, provided that the practice submits architects' plans and competitive tenders. Such plans:

- must be compliant with the Disability Discrimination Act 1995
- should have regard to the standards provided in *Primary and Social Care Premises: planning and design guidance* available at www.primarycare. nhsestates.gov.uk and
- should have regard to the minimum standards for practice premises as laid out in Schedule 1 of the Directions.

Any practice contemplating developing premises is advised to have dis-cussions with their LMC and the PCO before incurring professional fees in preparing a bid for premises monies.

Improvement grants

Improvement grants ranging in value from 33% to 66% of the project costs are now available subject to PCO budgetary constraints for the following items to support the delivery of primary medical services:

- extensions and enlargements of premises
- improving access to comply with the Disability Discrimination Act 1995
- improving lighting, ventilation or heating systems
- reasonable extension of telephone systems
- provision of car parking
- adaptations to meet the needs of children, the elderly, or the infirm
- improvements to security, and fire precaution compliance.

Generally, improvement grants are not used on leasehold premises because the GP does not own the premises.

Improvement grants are discretionary within budgetary constraints of the PCO and they cannot be used to procure land or buildings, repair, restore or maintain buildings. In deciding whether or not to grant an improvement grant the PCO must:

- consult the LMC
- satisfy itself that the proposal is value for money
- satisfy itself that it will support the delivery of GMS
- ensure that the development meets the design standards set out in guidance.

Applications must be supported where appropriate by architects' plans, relevant planning and building regulations consents. Building work requires three written quotes and the PCO must agree with the practice which quote represents the best value for money. The professional costs of architects' and surveyors' fees are now reimbursable together with VAT at the relevant rate. Project management fees are also reimbursable together with VAT in the case of TPD leaseback projects, together with the legal fees incurred in arranging the lease.

A common problem with premises funding has been that the once-in-a-lifetime capital spend on premises had to be funded within the year by the PCO. Consequently, many projects failed to proceed simply because their critical financial mass was too great for a single PCO to manage. Other reasons for failure to win funds were worthy projects that repeatedly missed out on funding by always coming second when competing for cash-limited funds. To obviate these problems the funds for premises developments will be held by a lead PCO for each Strategic Health Authority in England.

Expediting the process: dealing with initial costs

There are several chicken-and-egg situations that can arise upon disposal of existing premises. To resolve the problems associated with the disposal of existing practice properties, a number of flexibilities and discretionary funding streams are available through PCOs under the premises funding Directions. These problems frequently arise in localities where property values are low in relation to costs and such areas frequently have numbers of small practices in substandard premises. The flexibilities include:

- for practice removal to new approved *leasehold* premises

- grants to cover up to 100% of negative equity in old premises realised upon sale of the premises or
- mortgage redemption fees or
- grants to cover loans taken out to cover mortgage redemption fees or negative equity.

Other flexibilities applicable in situations where the move is to either owner-occupied or leasehold premises are denoted below and are subject to specific conditions and prior agreement with the PCO. Grants may be made:

- to reconvert old surgery premises to residential use by a registered social landlord
- towards the costs of surrendering or reassigning a lease
- towards the costs of stamp duty land tax.

For practitioners moving to new modern leasehold or owner-occupied premises, the following conditions apply.

- PCOs will not cover deficits caused by payment holidays and will offset from any payment gains arising through differentials between cost rent received and loan repayments.
- Borrowings incorporated in the surgery mortgage not connected with the land purchase, building or extension costs of the old premises are not covered.

Payments made under the scheme are subject to the following conditions:

- They are paid direct to the lender and not to the doctor.
- Negotiations with lenders must have occurred to minimise deficits and redemption charges.
- Alternative uses for premises must have been explored, including outline planning consents being obtained to improve their value and saleability.
- A businesslike approach must be taken to the sale of the outgoing premises to reduce the cost to the NHS.
- Sale of the premises must be on an open market basis and at arm's length not involving relatives or employees of the doctor or of the TPD.

Continuing the process: leasehold or rented premises

Once occupied, surgery premises incur ongoing capital and revenue costs. Leased premises can receive the lower of the actual lease rent plus VAT or the current market rent (CMR). The district valuer determines the CMR. In areas of poor property values, the PCO may increase the amount it will pay to ensure sufficient capital return to support new capital investment in premises. Where a developer provides certain equipment and furnishings as part of the lease in a modern set of premises, these too may be reimbursed.

Continuing the process: owner-occupied premises

The principle behind the Directions is to reimburse within defined limits the borrowing costs of purchasing, building or significantly refurbishing practice premises. The following costs are eligible components for which borrowing costs will be reimbursed in connection with building new premises or significant refurbishment:

- site purchase
- building works
- reasonable architect, surveyor and legal costs
- rolled up interest on loans taken out to procure the premises
- local authority and planning application fees
- fitting out and equipment costs
- VAT and stamp duty land tax.

Calculating borrowing costs: the prescribed percentage

Calculations are based upon the Bank of England published rates:

- fixed interest rate loans – the 20-year high gilt rate plus 1.5%
- variable rate loans – the Base Interest Rate plus 1%.

If you fund the premises without recourse to borrowing, then the PCO determines what rates will be paid and clearly specialist accountancy advice will need to be obtained.

Borrowing costs will be paid monthly until the loan is paid off. The amount payable to cover borrowing costs is calculated annually on the basis described above and paid in 12 equal instalments on the last day of the month. The process is repeated until either the loan is paid off, or the loan is renegotiated at a lower rate of interest, or until the practice elects to change to notional rent payments. Once a loan is paid off, conversion to notional rent is mandatory. If receiving borrowing costs upon a fixed interest rate basis, it is a condition of the payment that the PCO is notified if the lender changes or there is a reduction on the interest rate on the loan.

Notional rent payments

Notional rent, subject to conditions, is paid for premises used for provision of NHS general practice. Where a practice has been in receipt of borrowing costs reimbursement and makes an application to convert to notional rent, the PCO is compelled to accept the application and make notional rent payments. If there is no change in the use of the premises or no further capital investment in the premises, the notional rent is reviewed triennially.

Where the NHS has contributed capital to a building or refurbishment project at any time after 18 September 2003 the notional rent is abated for 10 years on a proportional basis as laid out in the Directions.

If a contractor in receipt of borrowing costs reimbursement makes further capital investments in the premises which result in a current market rent – and therefore a notional rent – lower than the payments made under the borrowing cost arrangements, a notional rent supplement can be made according to the formula in the Directions.

Premises operating costs

The following are reimbursable by PCOs for all types of premises:

- business rates
- water and sewerage charges
- clinical waste removal charges (subject to a value for money test on the contractor).

Where GPs lease premises with a service charge agreement the following items are allowed *if included* in the service charge agreement:

- gas and electricity charges
- insurance costs
- internal repair costs
- external repair costs
- buildings and ground maintenance charges.

It is by no means certain that landlords will agree any or all of these components in an agreement and legal advice is necessary. The amounts actually reimbursed will be abated in accordance with the Directions to prevent double reimbursement, as such costs are also reimbursed to GPs via other funding streams.

Premises standards

Minimum standards are now set out in the Directions for surgery premises. Where premises fail to meet the minimum standards, the PCO may issue a remedial notice giving six months for the practice to put things right. Before it issues a remedial notice, the PCO is required to consult the Local Medical Committee. Failure by a practice to take action will result in suspension of premises payments.

Transitional arrangements

During the switchover from the Red Book to the new GMS contract, some practices may temporarily utilise the default contract process because the legal basis for payments under the Red Book ceases on 31 March 2004. Effectively, the current payments continue on a no detriment basis during the transitional process.

Further reading

- *The National Health Service (General Medical Services – Premises Costs) (England) Directions 2004* which are made under The National Health Service Act 1977
- *The Future of GP Practice Premises: guidance for GPs.* Available at www. bma.org.uk.
- *Primary and Social Care Premises: planning and design guidance.* Available at www.primarycare.nhsestates.gov.uk.
- The Disability Discrimination Act 1995:
  - *A Guide for Everybody* – DL160
  - *What Service Providers Need to Know* – DL150
  - *What Employers Need to Know* – DL170.

GPC guidance notes are available at www.bma.org.uk on the following topics:

- *Practice Premises: Service Charge Agreements*
- *Partnership Agreements: guidance for GPs*
- *Surgery Premises: their valuation and an introduction to the rent and rates scheme*
- *Cost Rent Scheme: guidance for GPs*
- *Primary Care Trusts: a guide to estates and facilities matters.*

Department of Health publications are available at www.dh.gov.uk/publicationsandstatistics/publications/publicationslibrary/fs/en.

Chapter 13

Practice management

Peter Holden

Summary

- Practices now have much more flexibility to run their practices, including the staffing configuration to deliver the services they have contracted to provide. This will require a more businesslike approach to running the practice.
- The role of practice manager has evolved into a fully-fledged management role.
- There are three levels of role competency: administrative, managerial and strategic.
- There are nine core competency areas: practice operation and development, risk management, partnership issues, patient and community services, finance, human resources, premises and equipment, IM&T and population care.

A key feature of the new GMS contract is the release of practices from the suffocating and cloying bureaucracy of the old contract which required doctors to seek permission and funding for more staff time. From now on general practitioners must decide for themselves the skill mix of both clinical and administrative staff and the relative and absolute quantities of each type of staff to be employed.

Practices will need to adopt a business-like approach to their activities and ensure proper professional control, ethical and contractual oversight and financial profitability of *all* their activities, particularly those falling outside Essential and Additional Services. Failure to do so will have significant financial and professional consequences for practices and the equity-sharing partners in particular. No longer are specifically earmarked payments made for individual activities but overall payments encompass a range of activities. This is the only way to free up practices from the deluge of paperwork and heavy-handed control which became the hallmark of the old GMS contract, so redolent of its 1940s command and control philosophy. With the freedoms have come managerial responsibilities.

The consequences of such responsibilities are that the role of practice manager has evolved into a fully-fledged management role, encompassing elements of:

- general management
- financial management
- facilities management
- personnel management, including staff appraisal and training
- service planning and analysis
- business planning
- strategic planning
- maintenance of excellent working relationships with the PCO and LMC (or equivalents)
- negotiating with PCOs and Trusts
- GMS contract administration and compliance
- specific responsibility for achievement of the practice management component of the Quality and Outcome Framework
- acquaintance of relevant legislation, for example The National Health Service (General Medical Services Contracts) Regulations 2004 and The National Health Service (General Medical Services – Premises Costs) Directions 2004 (or their Welsh, Scottish and Northern Ireland counterparts)
- thorough working knowledge of the Standard General Medical Services Contract, the Statement of Financial Entitlements and the Department of Health document *Delivering Investment in General Practice: Implementing the New GMS Contract*.

It is unlikely that, except in a large practice, there will be sufficient resources to remunerate the calibre of individual who possesses all the above roles. It is possible for a practice to buy in specific expertise from outside agencies including the PCO or to form collaborative arrangements with other practices in a skill/competency sharing arrangement. In some practices the manager will be so crucial to the successful operation of the practice that it may be desirable to secure the loyalty and commitment of the manager by offering a partnership to them. The superannuation rules have been altered to permit this and for the manager as a non-clinician to remain in the NHS superannuation scheme.

The breadth and depth of practice management skills

Managers like all of us have professional strengths, interests and weaknesses. The competency framework for managers is laid out on pages 86 to 98 of the first contract document *The New GMS Contract 2003: Investing in General Practice*. A summary is provided below.

There are nine core competency areas, each broken down into topics. Each topic has three levels of role competency: administrative, managerial and strategic.

At the administrative competency level a manager knows how to collect and supply information on a given topic and has a basic understanding of what is being undertaken and why.

At the managerial competency level the manager has a full understanding of the process as it applies to the practice, is able to synthesise arguments and analyse and apply the data on a topic and collaborate with the GPs in planning or enacting change on an intra-practice basis.

At the strategic competency level the manager is fully conversant with a topic, able to review, revise and advise on the subject and has the competency, skills, knowledge, experience and credibility to advise other practices/the PCO on the way forward in topic development through, for example, feasibility/pilot studies. Such managers would have the credibility to lead changing practice on a topic not only at an intra-practice level but also at an inter-practice level.

The nine core competency areas of practice management and their component topics

1 **Practice operation and development**
- PCO meetings
- Development planning and report creation
- Clinical service provision
- Care Pathways
- Secondary and tertiary care liaison
- Strategy formulation
- Innovations
- Clinical audit
- Organisational audit

- Clinical effectiveness and evidence-based practice
- Resource allocation
- Professional development
- Research

2 Risk management

- Health and safety
- Fire safety
- Risk assessment
- Significant event reporting and audit
- Infection control
- Confidentiality
- Ethics
- Occupational health
- Poor performance
- Disaster planning

3 Partnership issues

- GP time management
- Locums
- Partnership meetings
- Partnership agreement
- Partnership changes
- Taxation
- Continuing professional development

4 Patient and community services

- Reception services
- Practice information
- Clinics/health promotion/Quality and Outcomes Framework (QOF)
- Complaints
- Community liaison
- Patient protection
- Community nursing liaison
- Social services liaison
- Working partnerships with rest of NHS
- Networking with managers from other practices

5 Finance

- Petty cash management
- Payroll and pensions
- Invoice payment

- Insurance
- Monthly accounting reconciliation processes
- Annual accounts
- Claims, targets, QOF payments
- Partnership drawings
- Quarterly list, Minimum Practice Income Guarantee or Global Sum reconciliation
- Banking and accountancy liaison
- Cash flow and budgeting
- Staff funding and budgeting
- Financial planning
- Service budgets
- Service deficiency reporting
- Resource negotiation

6 Human resources

- Staff management
- Staff meetings
- Rotas, work patterns, and European Working Time Directives
- Recruitment and staff selection
- Induction and training
- Employment practice
- Discipline and grievance procedures
- Performance review and staff appraisal
- Pastoral care

7 Premises and equipment

- Supplies, stock control, cash flow efficiencies and procurement
- Equipment monitoring, maintenance, replacement and procurement
- Facilities management
- Security
- Project management of equipment or premises

8 Information management and technology

- Patient record, data entry, good practice
- Data management, searches and reports
- Data security
- Data interpretation and manipulation
- Hardware maintenance and service contracts
- Oversee GP electronic links
- Crisis management, resolution and data recovery
- Project management of new systems and features

9 Population care
- Health needs assessment
- Service performance review
- Strategic delivery planning
- Service prioritisation
- Resource negotiation

From the above list of competencies it is clear that the intention behind the new contract is not only to professionalise and enhance the role of a practice manager but also to recognise the responsibilities devolved to practices as part of a 'high trust, low bureaucracy' contract. It is also clear that the intent over time is to develop practice managers who can deal with most tactical issues, leaving doctors time to think about the strategic direction of the practice and, of course, to do what they are trained to do: clinical medicine. Doctors should not be afraid of relinquishing tactical managerial roles to other trained professionals, as such individuals can often perform the task better than the well-meaning amateur with insufficient time to think through a problem. A well-run practice leaves the doctor with their mind uncluttered and unstressed, allowing concentration to be devoted to the clinical task in hand. Remember, you still have the final say, if you must, and this managerial delegation is no more an abrogation of responsibility than asking the nurse to manage a leg ulcer.

Practice manager and practice staff funding

The old rules of 70% reimbursement of two whole-time-equivalent ancillary staff per GP principal have disappeared. Indeed, over recent years, there has been a tendency for PCOs to devolve staff budgets to practices each year and there has been some variation in the exact percentage of direct reimbursement actually received by individual practices. However, under the old GMS contract, underspent staff budgets were usually clawed back through one means or another by PCOs. Under the new GMS contract any under- or overspends are to the practice's benefit or liability.

The new GMS Global Sum (and where applicable Minimum Practice Income Guarantee) contains within it the relevant staff funding from the baseline 12-month period ending 30 June 2003 and should cover any additional staff funding posts from 1 July 2003 to 1 April 2004. These monies are uplifted to April 2004 levels and have the extra employers' NHS superannuation contributions added. Practice staff costs in relation to the delivery of Essential and Additional Services are part of the Global Sum (or MPIG) allocation from which the practice will have to pay the employers' superannuation and National Insurance costs. Also within the Global Sum/MPIG are the monies for general staff training and professional updating of staff on professional matters except for Information Technology.

For Global Sum and MPIG practices, the Global Sum allocation incorporates a market forces factor weighting for staff costs for your area. It is, therefore, fully open to the discretion of the partnership within the terms of its contract with the PCO and subject to relevant legal obligations as to how, in what manner, it chooses to employ the quantity and type of staff and at what salary scale. This requires excellent practice management skills with human resources expertise.

It is incumbent upon practices when considering bidding for any Enhanced Service, whether local or national, to cost out the provision of services by the practice very carefully. The costing must include staff costs associated with such work because they are not specifically included in Global Sum/MPIG income streams and are not cross-subsidised by other activity.

It is very important that practices, particularly managers and managing partners, understand fully the concepts and practice of building and costing the business case for such Enhanced Services, as well as the more obvious clinical case. It is vital to practice partners' financial arrangements that this is done accurately. Otherwise a practice will not simply end up working for no reward but at a financial loss to the equity partners, who will be subsidising the NHS from their own pockets.

Chapter 14

The role of the Local Medical Committee

John Chisholm

Summary

- Under the new GMS contract the role of LMCs will be analogous to their existing role.
- The LMC has a wide variety of roles including being consulted by PCOs, becoming involved with issues on which practices or PCOs seek their support, and performing a representative function.
- The areas in which they will be involved include the planning and provision of services, patient list arrangements, the annual review process for the Quality and Outcomes Framework, contractual arrangements between PCOs and practices, and dispute resolution procedures.
- The existing financial arrangements for supporting LMCs will broadly continue.

The Local Medical Committee is one of the most enduring organisations in the UK healthcare system. LMCs precede the establishment of the National Health Service; indeed, they were first introduced in 1911 as part of Lloyd George's National Insurance Act, to give a local representative voice to GPs.

Throughout the UK, LMCs are the local structures that represent GPs. In England and Wales they have statutory, representative and pastoral functions. In Northern Ireland, they have not previously had statutory recognition, but will have under the new contract. In Scotland, the statutory functions are discharged by the GP Subcommittee of the Area Medical Committee, which in the majority of Board areas has a virtually identical constitution to the LMC for the same area.

The LMC is recognised as the voice for all General Medical Services GPs, whereas Personal Medical Services GPs and non-principal GPs have had to choose whether to pay a levy to their LMC. The position for non-principal GPs employed by a practice will change as a result of the practice-based nature of the new GMS contract.

Under the old Red Book GMS contract, there were numerous references to the LMC's role in the Regulations, Terms of Service and the Red Book itself, in England, Wales and Northern Ireland. In Scotland, those roles were undertaken by the GP Subcommittee. The new GMS contract will certainly involve the LMC (or its equivalent in Scotland) at least as closely. The contract document *The New GMS Contract 2003: Investing in General Practice* states that 'the role of LMCs (and their equivalents) and GP Subcommittees of Area Medical Committees under the new contract arrangements will be analogous to their existing role in each of the four countries'. Thus the new contract involves the LMC in a wide variety of roles; the PCO is variously required to consult the LMC, to inform the LMC or to include LMC representation, whilst on other issues either the PCO or a local practice can ask for the LMC's involvement and support. These roles and responsibilities are summarised in the rest of this chapter; in Scotland, some roles will be undertaken by the GP Subcommittee and some by the LMC.

Service provision

The Primary Care Organisation (PCO) must involve and consult LMCs about the planning and provision of services, the development and consideration of proposals for changing how those services are provided, and decisions affecting the operation of those services. One example where this consultation must take place is the obligation to discuss with the LMC first any PCO proposal to become a large-scale provider of primary medical services. Another is when the PCO is making commissioning decisions about securing essential primary medical services, in areas of historic underprovision, or when a surgery no longer delivers Essential Services, for instance when a single-handed GP has retired.

One crucial role for the LMC is in the categorisation of a service as an Enhanced Service. The PCO should inform the LMC about its proposals for commissioning Enhanced Services and agree with the LMC which of those services will count against the Local Enhanced Services spending floor. That local process is an essential component of the Technical Steering Committee's role in monitoring whether the expected amount has been spent, PCO by PCO and country by country.

When proposals for Local Enhanced Services are being developed in response to local need and specifications are being discussed between the PCO and local practices, either the practice or the PCO can ask the LMC (or its equivalent) for support.

The LMC is also involved in the new arrangements for list closure. When an assessment panel is convened to consider a contractor's application to close its list which has been rejected by the PCO, or convened to consider assigning patients to practices with closed lists, an LMC representative from a neighbouring Committee sits on the panel. When a PCO wants to assign patients to contractors with closed patient lists and refers its proposals to the panel, it has to notify the LMC that it has referred the matter.

The PCO must consult the LMC before refusing to grant approval of a proposal for out-of-hours arrangements. The PCO cannot withdraw its approval without consulting the LMC, except where immediate withdrawal is required in the interests of contractors and patients, in which case the PCO must notify the LMC.

Quality and Outcomes Framework

Either contractors or PCOs can choose to involve the LMC in the practice's annual review process. There are also two situations in which the LMC must be consulted if the PCO is considering rescoring a practice's quality points:

- if during the review visit there are questions about the accuracy of a practice's data and satisfactory remedial action has not taken place
- if the PCO has evidence that a contractor has been systematically and inappropriately referring patients to secondary care in order to maximise quality achievement points.

Contracts

PCOs should inform LMCs about local variations to practice contracts and the establishment of new practices. An LMC representative can be involved in the annual contract review if either the PCO or the practice wishes.

When contract breaches or failures arise, the LMC is involved. When a PCO is issuing a breach notice or a remedial notice where it believes a contractor is in default of its contractual obligations, the LMC should be consulted before the notice is issued. A PCO or a practice can invite the LMC to be involved in discussions about resolving a contract breach or failure.

The LMC is also involved in certain circumstances if a contract is being terminated:

- if the contractor no longer satisfies the provider conditions because the only GP contractor has left suddenly
- if a partnership change is considered to impact on the PCO's or practice's ability to fulfil the contract
- after an acrimonious partnership split.

A PCO may serve notice terminating the contract immediately if the contractor no longer satisfies the conditions set out in the Act and the Contract Regulations. If the contractor changes so that it no longer includes a GP and the doctor was part of a partnership and leaves it suddenly, the PCO can allow the contract to continue for up to six months. In such a case, the PCO must immediately consult the LMC.

If the PCO believes a partnership change is likely to have a serious impact on the contractor's or the PCO's ability to perform its obligations under the contract, the PCO can serve notice terminating the contract. Where practical, any such notice should follow consultation with the LMC; where that is not practical, the LMC should nonetheless be notified.

When a sudden or acrimonious change in the structure of the partnership occurs, the PCO may be unable to determine which of the remaining partners has a right to retain the contract. In such a situation, the PCO may serve notice terminating the contract. Again, where practical, any such notice should follow consultation with the LMC, and where not practical, notification of the LMC.

The PCO should inform the LMC about practice splits. The LMC should also be consulted on the process of arranging contracts: for individual GPs following a practice split, or following the retirement of a single-handed practitioner, or when a greenfield site practice is required.

The PCO should also consult the LMC before refusing a permanent contract to the holder of a temporary contract.

Dispute resolution and appeals

Either the PCO or the practice can request the presence and assistance of the LMC in conciliation during the process of dispute resolution. When non-contractual appeals by a practice about a disputed PCO decision are being addressed at local level, the PCO local review panel can include an LMC-appointed member.

Other issues

LMCs will consider complaints made to them by any medical practitioner against a GP contractor, and report the outcome of their consideration to the PCO if there are concerns relating to the efficiency of services provided under a contract. LMCs will also make arrangements for the medical examination of a GP contractor, where there are concerns that the doctor is incapable of adequately providing services under the contract. The LMC considers the report of such an examination and itself reports on the doctor's capability to the doctor, the contractor and the PCO.

The PCO is under a new legal obligation to develop and seek to agree with the LMC a suitable local policy for locum cover and payment arrangements.

Where a PCO is investigating alleged excessive prescribing by a contractor, it will consult the LMC about the allegations.

When the PCO is inspecting practice premises to assess compliance with the minimum quality standards, the visiting team includes an LMC representative. If a PCO branch surgery visit highlights shortcomings in premises standards, the LMC should be consulted.

The LMC should also be consulted about the local arrangements for implementing appraisal. Discussion with the LMC is required concerning the proportion of remediation costs that are to be met by the Workforce Development Confederation (or its equivalent).

One way of supporting remote rural practices is through twinning arrangements. Where twinning is a feasible option and is supported by the LMC, the PCO will do its utmost to support the implementation of twinning.

LMC funding

In broad terms, the existing arrangements for the financial support of LMCs will continue. It is only in Northern Ireland that the status of the LMC is changing, through the introduction of statutory recognition. The PCO will continue to collect levies, although the practice-based nature of the contract will be reflected in the manner in which levies are calculated and collected.

Conclusion

There are a great many functions for LMCs in relation to the new contract. Some of those functions are carried over from the old Red Book contract, while others are newly introduced. This extensive involvement of the LMC, together with the continuing need for a strong local voice for NHS general practitioners, undoubtedly means that Local Medical Committees will continue to endure, thrive and evolve in the future, just as they have for most of the last century.

Chapter 15

General practice as a career

Brian Dunn

Summary

The new GMS contract facilitates flexible working for GPs throughout their careers. It recognises the changes that have happened since the foundation of the NHS, the changes in the GP workforce and the expectations of young doctors contemplating a career in general practice. Major changes are:

- the ending of hours of availability
- salaried service
- opportunities for skills development and special interest development
- clinical leadership recognised as of equal value to clinical work
- development of teaching role in general practice
- improved seniority to reward experience
- improved pensions for GPs.

Introduction

There are a number of reasons why a change in the career structure for GPs has been sought.

- Since 1990, general practice has become a less popular career choice. Many junior doctors are spurning general practice for a career in hospital medicine because hospital doctors have a definite career path and salaries are often in excess of many general practitioners.
- The fluctuation in property prices made the risks of owning health centres much greater, leading to reluctance from new partners to commit themselves to the financial risks. Many general practitioners do not wish to have

the responsibilities of self-employed principals, staffing issues and the business side of general practice.

- Medical graduates are now predominantly female, their numbers in general practice are increasing and it is likely that, in the future, general practice will become a predominantly female profession.
- The concept of working for one practice for the rest of your working life has also become much less common, with GPs moving practices – sometimes several times.
- As the 1990s progressed, because of increased patient expectation, poor investment in primary care, undervaluing of GPs and seemingly constant organisational change, morale in British general practice plummeted, leading to many experienced GPs opting for early retirement and younger GPs switching to other specialties or leaving the profession altogether.
- The recruitment and retention crisis led to a further drop in GP morale and with principals' positions increasingly difficult to fill, many practices dealing with a failure to replace a partner closed their lists to new patients, resulting in PCOs allocating patients to practices that were already having difficulty coping with their present patient list.

The new GMS contract promised GPs that it would:

- facilitate the introduction of a new career structure
- support the introduction of protected time for skills development
- enable the widespread employment of salaried GPs in GMS where this best suits practice and practitioner preferences
- deliver family-friendly improvements
- encourage recruitment and retention through national schemes such as golden hello schemes, sabbatical schemes, flexible career schemes and returners schemes
- support the development of practice staff including nurses and managers.

One of the longer term measures the new GMS contract promotes is flexibility for GPs to develop a modular approach to career development, responding to the needs of their patients, their own interests and aptitudes and the complementary interests and skills of their partners.

Skills development

The flexibility of the new GMS contract allows GPs to broaden their clinical experience and enables them to work in a range of clinical settings to develop new skills. This opportunity may be taken up by newly trained GPs and those returning after a career break, but may also be used by experienced GPs to improve their clinical care in general practice and widen the range of services they can offer patients in the primary care setting. GPs, some remaining active in their practice, others taking leave of absence for a period, will be enabled (with the agreement of their partners) to take up salaried posts in a hospital specialty without detriment to their income or pension. They will be trained in skills normally only available in secondary care. These services may be resourced as Enhanced Services and PCOs will be able to use the skills of such GPs to enhance primary care and reduce pressures on the secondary sector. GPs are generalists and most wish to remain so, but many GPs have now developed a special interest – not because they are frustrated specialists but because the special interest helps them and their practice to deliver a high quality service to their patients.

Special interest development

GPs have never had a career structure. GP training became established in the 1970s and mandatory around 1980. The lack of a career structure meant that when a GP joined a practice and progressed to a parity share of profits, they continued to work with only annual increments in their pay. Many GPs continued to practise in a medical specialty as hospital practitioners or clinical assistants. These posts were not well remunerated and were carried on by GPs because of their interest and the professional satisfaction gained.

This contract will allow GPs to pursue clinical interests within primary care. GPs have experienced a transfer of work from the secondary to primary sector over the past 20 years. This work has been largely unresourced and has added to the work stresses of practices. Many GPs are prepared to accept this work and to look at other areas where they may accept work that has traditionally been carried out in secondary care. The Enhanced Services area of the contract provides a framework for resourcing this work and allowing GPs to extend their training and skills to provide services generally not available in primary care.

These services may include those set out in the National Enhanced Services list or other services according to the interests and training of the GPs. The services may be offered to patients of their own practice or may include other patients from other practices if contracted by the PCO.

The GP with a Special Interest (GPwSI) has become popular with Government and the Royal College of General Practitioners has produced guidance on training and the delivery of these services within primary care. Special interests include more specialised minor surgery, more specialised chronic disease management, endoscopy and orthopaedic/rheumatology assessment and injection clinics.

Not all of the special interests will be clinical. Many GPs are involved in education (GP registrars and medical students), clinical trials, PCO management roles, occupational health, journalism, LMC and GPC work.

All these developments are further supported by the move to practice-based contracts, with the practice determining the appropriate skill mix, making the best use of other professions and staff, including the development of practice management competencies (*see* Chapter 13).

Clinical leadership

This phase of a GP's career is more likely to be in the later stages – although it is not always and is certainly not necessarily expected to be. Some GPs at the start of their career will have had experience of medico-politics at a local or national level or in research. These GPs may wish to start their career after completing training with a reduced clinical commitment and pursue their other interests. Activities in this section include clinical roles, PCO work, LMC work, appraisal and clinical governance leads. The contract recognises that non-clinical work can be rewarding and as important as the clinical component – easing the process for many GPs who in the past have had to put pressures on their partners and frequently can only carry out these tasks by imposing on their long-suffering partners' patience and sometimes shouldering an extra burden of clinical work or dissatisfaction from patients at the unavailability of their doctor.

The new GMS contract affects not just clinical but also organisational standards. Some of these organisational standards such as those in the Quality and Outcomes Framework – while being worthy – are voluntary. Others such as clinical governance and appraisal are mandatory and all GPs must participate with support from the PCO. Many GPs will have commitments as appraisers and clinical governance leads in the PCO.

The salaried option

The new GMS contract has made great strides forward in developing national model terms and conditions of service for salaried GPs. These terms and conditions will be a requirement of contractors for new appointees as part of the new Standard GMS Contract and PCO-employed GPs can expect the new terms and conditions of service to apply to them as well. Although this will create financial pressures for some practices as small businesses, good employment practice must be encouraged and PCOs should support practices financially where this is required. Practices that particularly focus on achieving high employment standards may also be eligible for seeking 'Improving Working Lives' accreditation.

With the development of portfolio careers, it is the intention to try to ensure easy entry and exit between self-employed and salaried GP options so that GPs may tailor their contractual status to suit their career development.

Appraisal

Funding for appraisal is included in the Global Sum from 1 July 2004. Appraisal is a formative and confidential process and it has the potential to facilitate professional development for all GPs and will form a large part of the requirements for GPs to be revalidated by the General Medical Council. The present intention is that GPs must have an annual appraisal but additional information about their performance may be required from their clinical governance lead.

Appraisal is a useful tool, providing protected time for GPs to assess their performance, look at what they have done over the previous year and plan their continuing professional development for the next year to assist them to perform better. It is not a pass/fail system and is not a tool to recognise under-performance. The success of appraisal will depend on the quality of training of the appraisers and it is essential that remuneration rates will be adequate to attract appraisers in sufficient numbers to allow all GPs to participate in the process.

Teaching role

Teaching of medical students has traditionally been carried out in hospitals with short attachments to general practice. In recent years, with better premises, increased range of services and increasing pressures on hospital staff, more of this undergraduate training has taken place in general practice. Some practices, especially those close to universities, can look forward to a greater involvement in undergraduate training and closer links with the university.

GP training is likely to change in future years – some of the suggestions are a longer training period, attachment to a practice for the duration of training, shorter periods in hospital specialties (three or four months instead of six) and a longer period training in a practice. These changes may lead to greater opportunities for GPs to spend a greater proportion of their time in education and the contract will facilitate this.

Seniority payments

GP seniority payments in the old contract depended on two factors – the number of years qualified and the number of years as a GP principal. The payments were in step with a substantial rise between the stages. The system disadvantaged those doctors that had spent longer periods in hospital medicine or worked for several years as a GP locum. The new seniority scheme delivers a 30% increase in resources by 2005–06. It abolishes the requirement of number of years as a principal and introduces the concept of 'reckonable service'. To qualify for seniority payments, GPs must be in post for at least two years and the reckonable service is then calculated from the date of first registration (provisional registration). Only public sector clinical service is reckonable and service in other EEA states is reckonable. GPs who have worked as GP locums can have this service counted if they can provide proof of their earnings in those years.

If a GP earns less than one third of the average GP superannuable income, they will not be eligible for seniority payments. GPs with superannuable income of between one third and two thirds of the average GP superannuable income will be eligible for 60% of the seniority payment based on their reckonable years. GPs with superannuable income of greater than two thirds will be eligible for the full award.

The seniority scheme is intended to encourage senior GPs to continue in practice and attract 'returners' – trained GPs who are not working or are working in other areas of the NHS or private sector.

Other retention initiatives

The current Flexible Careers Scheme, Retainers' Scheme and Returners' Scheme will continue and have not been changed as a result of the new GMS contract.

There was some talk about establishing sabbatical arrangements for GPs. In terms of determining a national model scheme, for example, no progress has yet been made. Nevertheless, some notional funding in England has been made available through the PCO-administered funding stream for PCOs to support local sabbatical programmes.

'Improving Working Lives'

Again, these Department of Health initiatives, including the delivery of the NHS childcare strategy into primary care, remain largely unchanged as a result of the new GMS contract. One difference is the introduction of a Directed Enhanced Service for services to violent patients, which puts the responsibility on the PCO to commission such services from an appropriate provider in secure facilities.

Flexible working and skill mix

The new GMS contract encourages practices to work flexibly using skill mix to the fore in order that the most appropriate person does the work. This may mean doctors delegating tasks to other health professionals and concentrating on tasks that only doctors can do. Many practices have begun this process. For others, it will be a culture shock, but those with concerns can learn from others. The contract allows GPs to control their workload, but without a change in attitude by many GPs, the benefits of this may be lost.

Case study

One practice that has embraced flexible working describes their model as follows:

- no GP should spend all their professional time doing only general practice
- GPs are overqualified for a lot of the work they do
- nurses and particularly nurse practitioners in certain circumstances can be more effective than doctors
- the role of the GP with Special Interest is cost-effective
- we try to delegate the work to the least expensive person who is safe to carry out the work.

We have nine partners, only one works as a 'full-time' nine-session partner and usually one or two of those sessions are administrative. The rest vary from eight down to four sessions per week.

We have two full-time nurse practitioners, a full-time and a part-time practice nurse, and are about to employ a healthcare assistant.

The nurse practitioners see presentations within their clinical competence. They do not use protocols but use skills learnt – as GPs do.

Except for diabetes, the nurse practitioners do no routine clinics – the practice nurses do this. The healthcare assistant will do all measurements including spirometry and data gathering, leaving the practice nurse to manage the condition and give advice.

To channel workload appropriately the nurse practitioners make almost all their own appointments – very few are available for booking by receptionists.

Whenever a patient phones for an appointment, they are offered the first opportunity available. If they feel it is more urgent, they are triaged by the nurse practitioner, who assesses the problem. There are six possible outcomes:

- advice only
- advice and a prescription – e.g. cystitis
- an appointment with the nurse practitioner
- an appointment with a GP the same day
- an appointment with a GP later
- go directly to A&E – injuries etc.

Pensions

The GP pension scheme based on lifetime earnings has traditionally been outperformed by the final salary scheme of consultants. Some elements of GP remuneration were fully superannuable and others were either partly superannuable or not included in the calculations of earnings for GP superannuation. The new GMS contract allows all NHS income to be superannuable. This will allow for a considerable uplift in GP pensions.

Intended Average Net Income determined by the Doctors and Dentists Review Body was used to determine the Uprating Factor of GP pensions. This will no longer exist and GP pensions will be based on total NHS profits of GPs. Because all NHS earnings will be reckonable for superannuable purposes, these earnings will include:

- all NHS profits from Global Sum, Enhanced Services and the Quality and Outcomes Framework
- all out-of-hours work for GP co-operatives
- profit from premises
- GP education
- statutory reports.

The Uprating Factor is calculated on a national basis and those GPs that do not own premises and do not participate in GP educational activities will benefit from the increased Uprating Factor.

Flexibilities have been introduced into the superannuation scheme to ensure that moving between independent contractor and employee status will no longer damage GP pensions.

Chapter 16

Pensions

Simon Fradd

Summary
- All NHS profits to be superannuated.
- Dynamising based on overall increase in GPs' superannuable income.
- Pension to be based on actual personal profits.
- Employers' contributions to be included in practice income.
- New flexibilities to protect against changes in employment status.

Superannuable income

The way in which GPs' pensions are calculated is unique in the NHS superannuation scheme. Whereas employed NHS staff have their pensions based on their final salary, our pension is based on lifetime earnings. Each year our superannuable income is added to a lifetime earnings pool and at retirement an Accrual Factor of 1.4% is applied to this final sum to calculate the pension payable. In addition a lump sum of three times the annual pension is paid on retirement. This lump sum is entirely tax free.

Table 16.1: Example of lump sum calculation

	£
Lifetime earnings	1 000 000
Pension 1.4%	14 000
Tax free lump sum	42 000

If no correction was made for annual pay awards, lifetime earnings would be seriously eroded by inflation over the years. Thirty years ago a GP only earned £4000 or £5000 a year. It is therefore essential to make an adjustment each year to the lifetime earnings amount to ensure that annual pay awards by the Doctors and Dentists Review Body are taken into account. Historically this has been done by applying an Uprating Factor (commonly known as the dynamising factor) equivalent to the annual uplift in fees and allowances.

Table 16.2: Example of Uprating Factor calculation

	£
Lifetime earnings	1 000 000
2002–03 Uprating Factor 9.0%	1 090 000

This mechanism is fundamentally sound. However, in 1990, when higher target payments for childhood immunisations and cervical screening came into existence, they were excluded from the Uprating Factor. Consequently pensions have not truly kept pace with inflation. Under the new GMS contract this will be corrected and the Uprating Factor will be further enhanced.

Calculating pensionable NHS pay

For self-employed GPs, profits are the result of NHS income less expenses. Under the Red Book the ratio of profit to expenses has been averaged across the profession. There were three classes of NHS revenue:

- *Group 1 Payments*: These are treated wholly as expenses. These include items such as reimbursed premises and staff costs.
- *Group 2 Payments*: These are treated as 100% profit. These include items such as seniority payments.
- *Group 3 Payments*: These are treated as partially profit and partially as reimbursement of expenses. The Technical Steering Committee[1] calculates this ratio each year from sampling GP tax returns. A fixed factor is then applied to all payments which fall under this head. Group 2 payments

---

[1] The Technical Steering Committee is a joint committee with professional statisticians, representatives of the GPC UK negotiating team, representatives from the four Departments of Health of the UK, and representatives from the NHS Confederation.

make up a large part of the NHS funding we receive, for instance Basic Practice Allowance and Item of Service Fees.

This system is inherently unfair. Individual NHS pensions do not reflect the actual profits of GPs. In addition, there are several elements of NHS income which are not currently taken into account in calculating our pensions. For example, profits from practice premises. These average £900 per year per GP.

Under the new system NHS superannuation will be based on the actual profits of each practice each year and will be allotted to individual partners according to their partnership agreement. This system means that actual pensionable income will not be known until the practice accounts have been finalised.

Superannuation contributions

Currently the Primary Care Organisation is responsible for paying the employer contribution of 7% for GP partners and individual partners are responsible for making the employee contribution of 6%. From 1 April 2004 the employer contribution is being increased to 14% in England and Wales.[2]

In future this employer contribution will be added to the money the practice receives and the practice will be responsible for payments. The reason for this is so that if colleagues reach the new Inland Revenue pensions cap they will be able to opt out of making further payments to the superannuation scheme but will keep the employer contribution. This represents an enhancement of 14% of profits. GPs will be free to do what they want with this money.

Each month the Primary Care Organisation will make a deduction on account of the superannuable contributions for both the employee and employer payments from the practice's revenue. It is anticipated that this amount will be equivalent to the contributions for the previous year's final superannuable income divided by 12.

When the practice has prepared their tax return for the financial year they will also complete a statement for the Pensions Agency. This is a very simple form and only includes data which colleagues will need available in order to complete their tax return. There should be no – or minimal – costs incurred in having your accountant complete it.

The practice will have to send a cheque with the return to cover the balance of superannuation contributions due.

---

[2] The employer contribution has not yet been determined for Scotland and Northern Ireland.

The annual return to the NHS Pensions Agency

It is essential that you include both NHS and non-NHS professional income and expenses in this return. The reason for this is that non-NHS expenses are proportionately much lower than for NHS work. If both sources of income and expenses are not shown your NHS pension will be much lower than it should be. In addition it will depress the national Uprating Factor.

This is how it works:

Table 16.3: Excluding non-NHS income and expenditure

	£	
NHS income	300 000	
NHS expenses		200 000
Total	300 000	200 000
NHS profits	100 000	

Table 16.4: Including non-NHS income

	£	
NHS income	300 000	
Non-NHS income	100 000	
NHS expenses		200 000
Non-NHS expenses		20 000
Total	400 000	220 000
Total profit	180 000	

$$\text{NHS profit} = \text{Total profit} \times \frac{\text{NHS Income}}{\text{Total Income}}$$

$$180\,000 \times \frac{300\,000}{400\,000} = 180\,000 \times 0.75 = 135\,000$$

Although this example is fairly extreme it illustrates how superannuation will be underestimated if all sources of income are not included. In this case the difference is between £100 000 and £135 000 or 35%!

Remember the effect on the Uprating Factor will be the same. We owe it to the whole profession to get our Pensions Return correct.

The Uprating or Dynamising Factor

In future the Uprating Factor will be based on the increase in the total NHS superannuable income of all GPs in the United Kingdom. As it has been agreed that all NHS income will be superannuable there will be no payments left out of the calculation as they have been in the past.

For 2004–05 the calculation will be:

$$\frac{\text{Total GP NHS Income in } 2004-05}{\text{Total GP NHS income in } 2003-04}$$

This is the only methodology that will ensure that in future the Uprating Factor truly reflects the income of the profession. However, there is one drawback. The calculation cannot be finalised until the total payments for superannuation have been received by the Pensions Agency. As has been explained above, this will not be until after GPs have filed their annual tax returns. The final Uprating Factor for any given year will not be available until 12 months after the end of the financial year. In other words for 2004–05 the final factor will be published in April 2006.

This is not as serious as it sounds. First, the factor is only relevant in the year of retirement. No money is paid out of the scheme until retirement or death, whichever comes first. Second, it has been agreed that each year the Technical Steering Committee will calculate an interim Uprating Factor to be used to calculate all payments until the final factor is available. At the latter time a supplement will be paid to doctors who have retired in the relevant year. This will cover both outstanding and ongoing pension payable and an addition to the lump sum.

The interim factor will be less than the final factor in order to avoid any clawback.

Flexibilities

All doctors have to undertake some hospital work before becoming principals in general practice. Before the introduction of mandatory vocational training it was possible to go straight into practice immediately after the pre-registration house officer year. Since 1983 everyone has had to do at least three additional years of vocational training. Throughout this time we are employees and the NHS pension is based on final salary. This is known as the 'officer' basis of calculation. In addition, posts such as a clinical assistant or hospital practitioner are also based on the officer method.

Under the Red Book doctors who had more than 10 years' officer service before becoming a GP principal or more than one year after becoming a principal were given two separate pensions on retirement. One was calculated on their lifetime earnings as a GP and the other on final salary as an officer. Because the Accrual Factor for officers is 1.25% and because the officer pension prior to retirement is linked to inflation rather than earnings, some doctors lost pension.

New flexibilities have been already introduced into the NHS superannuation scheme as a result of the new GMS contract. These are to ensure that no one suffers as a result of having a different lifetime earnings pattern from the average. In each case the best method of calculation will be used. GPs do not have to apply for the use of flexibilities.

GP principals with less than 10 years' pre-practitioner officer service

For this group of doctors the best of three alternative methods of calculating pension entitlement will be used at retirement:

1   separate pensions for GP and officer (for hospital work)
2   adding the hospital earnings pro-rata to GP earnings in order to calculate a single GP pension
3   dynamising hospital earnings in line with national increase in GP pay and adding this to lifetime dynamised GP earnings to calculate a single GP pension.

GP principals with more than 10 years' pre-practitioner officer service

For this group of doctors the better of two alternative methods of calculating pension entitlement will be used at retirement:

1 separate pensions for GP and officer (for hospital work)
2 dynamising hospital earnings in line with national increase in GP pay and adding this to lifetime dynamised GP earnings to calculate a single GP pension.

Added years

These will be added into the calculations as if they were effective at the date at which the added years contract was entered into.

Chapter 17

Private fees

Andrew Dearden

Summary
- The new GMS contract does not extend the opportunities for practices to charge patients.
- The previous exceptions to the ban on charging patients have been clarified.

The new GMS contract is specific about when GPs can charge patients. It does not go as far as many GPs would wish, but the Government is firmly opposed to introducing new charges to patients. The Contract Regulations specify the circumstances when GPs can levy charges and these are:

- from statutory bodies for the purpose of that body's statutory function
- from employers or schools for routine medical examinations
- for non-primary medical services in a nursing home
- for medico-legal examinations after RTAs
- for attending a police station to examine a detainee
- for preparing a variety of medico-legal reports
- for travel immunisations not remunerated under the contract
- for prescribing drugs for foreign travel
- for medical examination for exemption to wear a seatbelt.

Despite a number of attempts to expand and simplify the arrangements for charging patients private fees for non-GMS services, the Government is adamant that it will not extend the extant provisions. Thus, the opportunities for charging fees have remained largely untouched although a clarification has been achieved in a number of areas.

In this chapter we will look at the specific services that a GP may provide to their own patients, for which a fee may be charged. The list of these services is listed in Schedule 5 of the *National Health Service (General Medical Services Contract) Regulations 2004*. The Regulations state:

> *The contractor may demand or accept, directly or indirectly, a fee or other remuneration:*
> *(a) from any statutory body for services rendered for the purposes of that body's statutory function; ...*

Many statutory bodies need to ask for reports so they can fulfil their responsibilities. It does not matter what the underlying reason for the report is; reports done for this reason are subject to a fee being made by the GP. If the body is a statutory one, when they ask you for a report, you are in fact acting in the capacity of a medical advisor, which is not part of Essential or Additional Services, and so is not covered by the Global Sum or any other part of your GMS contract.

None of the work that falls under the collaborative arrangements falls within the definition of Essential or Additional Services. GPs have no contractual obligation (under GMS) to prepare the requested report.

Remember, however, that much of this work will now be classified as NHS work for superannuable purposes from April 2004. For example, DS1500 attendance allowance under special rules will be classified this way and so the fees charged will benefit you now and when you draw your pension.

> *(b) from any body, employer or school for a routine medical examination of persons for whose welfare the body, employer or school is responsible, or an examination of such persons for the purpose of advising the body, employer or school of any administrative action they might take; ...*

This has not changed from the old Red Book. It is helpful to have a practice policy and fee structure for this work. This section covers all schools and universities, which seem to ask for an increasing number and variety of forms and reports. The reason given for the report does not matter. Each one attracts a separate fee.

The organisation requesting the information is responsible for the fee. You can provide the patient with whatever you feel appropriate for their specific needs. For example, you could provide them with a simple private sick note, in the case of an absence of one or two days due to illness, or a full medical report if prolonged illness may have affected their attendance through the entire year. The choice of what level of report to provide should be made on clinical and not financial grounds. Some organisations may attempt to shift the expense of a report to the patient. This should be resisted by practices in order to deter requests for spurious and time-wasting reports.

> *(c) for treatment which is not primary medical services or otherwise required to be provided under the contract and which is given:*
> *(i) pursuant to the provisions of section 65 of the Act, or*

(ii) in a registered nursing home which is not providing services under that Act,

if, in either case, the person providing the treatment is serving on the staff of a hospital providing services under the Act as a specialist providing treatment of the kind the patient requires and if, within 7 days of giving the treatment, the contractor or the person providing the treatment supplies the Primary Care Trust, on a form provided by it for the purpose, with such information about the treatment as it may require; ...

Section 65 of the 1977 Act allows Health Authorities to make available at hospitals for which they are responsible accommodation and services for private patients who give undertakings to pay the appropriate charges.

This provision allows private fees to be charged if the contractor satisfies the qualifying test at the end of the clause.

(d) under section 158 of the Road Traffic Act 1988[1]; ...

Even though we have been able to charge for this in the past, most of us have not done so. If a patient attends on their own accord or is seen by you at the request of the police following a RTA, purely to have their injuries documented for entirely legal reasons, i.e. to enable you to produce a legal report later on, you are entitled to charge the patient a fee.

The key phrase is 'but not otherwise treating'. If they come to you for treatment of their injuries you cannot charge them for this. However, it is unlikely that you would record all of their injuries to the level of detail often required for a legal report when treating their injuries. You must make it clear to the patient that the recording of injuries sustained in the RTA for legal purposes incurs a charge, though the treatment of their injuries does not.

You should inform the patient of the charge before you proceed with the examination. If they refuse to pay, you are under no obligation to record their injuries as requested.

(e) when it treats a patient under regulation 24(3), in which case it shall be entitled to demand and accept a reasonable fee (recoverable in certain circumstances under regulation 24(4)) for any treatment given, if it gives the patient a receipt on a form supplied by the PCT with whom it holds a contract; ...

Regulation 24(3) allows fees to be charged to patients who apply for the provision of Essential Services and claim to be on the contractor's list of patients but cannot produce a medical card and where the contractor has reasonable doubts about the person's claim. If, however, the patient can

---

[1] 1988 c.52. Section 158 was amended by SI 1995/889, article 3.

subsequently satisfy the PCT that he/she was on the list of patients, the PCT can recover the fee from the contractor's income and pay it to the patient.

> *(f) for attending and examining (but not otherwise treating) a patient:*
> *(i) at his request at a police station in connection with proceedings which the police are minded to bring against him*
> *(ii) at the request of a commercial, educational or not-for-profit organisation for the purpose of creating a medical report or certificate*
> *(iii) for the purpose of creating a medical report required in connection with an actual or potential claim for compensation against any person that the patient and his legal advisers believe may have been responsible for some harm that the patient has suffered; ...*

This section makes it clear that, if you are asked by anyone, for example an employer, a commercial or not-for-profit company or an educational organisation, to attend and examine a patient solely for the purposes of producing a medical report, a charge can be made to the requesting person or persons. Attending and producing the report falls outside Essential Services so you are entitled to charge the requesting person or organisation. It is always worth making sure the requesting person knows that a separate fee is chargeable, and, if possible, is given some idea of the amount likely to be incurred.

> *(g) for treatment consisting of an immunisation for which no remuneration is payable by the Primary Care Trust and which is requested in connection with travel abroad; ...*

The fees attracted by the provision of this service have not changed under the new contract. Many practices maximise the income generated by these services by setting up travel clinics. This is something worth thinking about if you have not already done so.

There have been many queries as to whether the position on charging for some travel immunisations has changed. The plain answer is no. The travel immunisations that GPs could charge for under the old contract are the same as those they may charge for under the new contract, and there has been no extension to the list. The funding for travel vaccines that were paid for by the NHS through the Statement of Fees and Allowances has been mapped to the Global Sum funding stream. As this forms part of the Additional Service under the new GMS contract for adult immunisations and vaccinations, practices may opt out of providing this service at a cost of 2% of the practice's Global Sum being deducted. If a practice opts out of this service, they cannot charge patients for providing it privately.

> *(h) for prescribing or providing drugs or appliances (including a collection of such drugs and appliances in the form of a travel kit) which a patient requires to have in his possession solely in anticipation of the onset of an*

ailment or occurrence of an injury while he is outside the United Kingdom but for which he is not requiring treatment when the medicine is prescribed; ...

Increasingly, patients are asking for prescriptions for medication that they wish to take, or have been advised to take with them while travelling. This is not for current medical conditions but 'just in case they need them'. These medications can be provided to patients but should be prescribed on a private prescription for which a fee can be charged. Requested medications include, for example, drugs like loperamide or antibiotics in case of diarrhoea or antihistamines in case of insect bites.

This section now includes medical supplies as well as medications. If a patient requests you to supply them with a 'travel pack' (which may include supplies like needles and syringes), a charge can be made for this service. However, you must not make a charge on the patient for these travel packs from items which the NHS supplies you for free. You would either have to purchase the items and make up or purchase packs.

(i) for a medical examination:
(i) to enable a decision to be made whether or not it is inadvisable on medical grounds for a person to wear a seat belt, or
(ii) for the purpose of creating a report:
(aa) relating to a road traffic accident or criminal assault, or
(bb) that offers an opinion as to whether a patient is fit to travel; ...

Similar to (f) above, this service of producing a report for, or on behalf of, a patient is not part of GMS and so attracts a separate fee.

(j) where the person is not one to whom any of paragraphs (a), (b) or (c) of section 38(1) of the Act applies (including by reason of regulations under section 38(6) of that Act), for testing the sight of that person; ...

Very few GPs provide this service today, but it was left in for those who do.

(m) where it is a contractor which is authorised or required by a Primary Care Trust under regulation 20 of the Pharmaceutical Regulations to provide drugs, medicines or appliances to a patient and provides for that patient, otherwise than under pharmaceutical services, any Scheduled drug; ...

This allows for fees to be charged where a Black or Grey listed drug is supplied privately by a dispensing chemist.

(n) for prescribing or providing drugs for malaria chemoprophylaxis.

As more and more people travel to exotic climes, so the demand for this service continues to grow. You may charge a patient who, due to reasons of travelling, requires malaria prophylaxis. The drugs should be prescribed on a private prescription for which a charge can be made. The patient will then need to pay the chemist separately for the drugs.

Chapter 18

Special geographical circumstances

Peter Holden

Summary
- There are additional factors that need to be taken into account for general practice in specific geographical circumstances, particularly practices in remote, rural or isolated areas.
- The issues that particularly affect such practices include dispensing, minor injury services, community hospitals, out-of-hours services, branch surgeries, and immediate care and responder services.

The consequences of a surgery consultation: the geographical difference

General practice in the United Kingdom is a unique mixture of high standards of professional approach to general practice with different practices serving widely differing socio-economic groups under widely differing circumstances. By and large, whether a consultation is being conducted in an inner city consulting room or on a remote Scottish island, the essence of the consultation is the same. The clinical, diagnostic and inter-personal skills brought to the consultation part of patient services are largely the same wherever routine general practice consultations take place.

The logistical consequences from a consultation in a practice located in a conurbation and the general clinical management approach will be very different from that in a rural practice – for example, where a patient requires blood tests, an ECG or X-rays.

In an urban practice the logistical procedures may be limited to the issue of the appropriate request forms together with instructions as to which part of the hospital outpatient department the patient should attend in order to obtain the tests.

In a more rural or isolated practice, the patient may well have the blood samples taken at the surgery and may even have to:

1 return on another day or
2 go to a distant main surgery where there is
   – practice staff to undertake the procedure
   – a pathology courier service available.

In a remote practice, the doctor may have to obtain all the samples and record the ECG himself at that time, particularly in a domiciliary consultation situation, simply because of the distance or travelling time to the patient's home. This is despite having practice staff able to perform the tasks available at the surgery.

Special geographical circumstances

Remote, rural or isolated practices (which includes quite sizeable market town communities as well as islands) by virtue of their distance from secondary care have very different practising circumstances from those practices located in the larger centres of population. Such practices inevitably are unable to benefit from economies of scale. Some clinical management decisions are dictated by distance or transport availability.

Travelling time reduces efficiency of operation for professional staff and the doctors are often the only medical presence in a community. Because of this, rural, remote or isolated practices frequently have to provide a much broader range of services to their patients, partly because of tradition and patient expectation and partly because of the professional ethos required to both practise and live in a small community. Although there are many benefits to practising in special geographical circumstances, the demographic construction of rural populations and the expectations of younger doctors and more importantly their families mean that general practice under such circumstances is becoming unpopular and recruitment difficulties are compounding the workload issue.

Additional factors concerning general practice in special geographical circumstances

- The particular operational management skills for ordinary general practice.
- The logistical and organisational arrangements required to underpin the practice – for example, branch surgeries and near-patient testing.
- The requirement to be more involved in emergency care provision – for example, minor injuries and immediate care/first responder services.
- The requirement to undertake a broader range of clinical services within the practice – for example, more advanced minor surgery and near-patient testing.

Dispensing

Special geographical circumstances are not synonymous with the requirement to dispense. However, the obligation to dispense is much more common in such areas. Dispensing is not part of General Medical Services, so much so that the activity is governed by completely separate regulations. This NHS work is, however, additional to ordinary general practice and it is now remunerated separately from GMS funding.

The rules concerning who may dispense and the conduct of dispensing have not changed from the old GMS contract.

Minor injuries services

Many practices operating in special geographical situations have to provide a minor injuries service both in their surgery and also out of hours. This is very disruptive to practice routine. Such work is very unpredictable and frequently demands immediate attention. There are premises and staffing costs associated with such activities which are disproportionate to the practice list size. Until now such work has gone unrecognised both financially and professionally.

The Minor Injuries National Enhanced Service under the new GMS contract is a specification for an *in-hours only* minor injuries service. It is designed to resource and remunerate those practices where for special geographical reasons it is not possible or proper to send a patient to a distant A&E unit for minor matters. Full details of the specification are available in the supporting documentation to *The New GMS Contract 2003: Investing in General Practice*.

Value of the Minor Injuries NES

For provision of an in-hours Minor Injuries NES, the 2004–05 fee is a £1032.25 retainer plus £51.61 per patient episode. The PCO may wish to agree a cap that, as it is approached, will trigger discussions with the practice about the service. It should include an evaluation of the impact of the service in reducing demand on other parts of the service including the avoidance of ambulance transfers. If the cap is reached and there are insufficient funds, the practice should cease further minor injuries work until funds become available again. Indeed, this should be written into the original contract so that there can be no argument about having to give three months' notice of cessation of service.

Many practices in special geographical situations also staff the community hospital where minor injuries services can be provided and, although relieved of the logistical and facilities provision burdens of such services, the doctors still have to provide the clinical input, often at short notice on a 24/7 basis. Such work, by virtue of its unpredictable nature and its potential to occupy a doctor for a considerable length of time, does not lend itself to traditional cover by out-of-hours co-operative arrangements.

Community hospitals

Almost 4000 GPs staff nearly 400 community hospitals, providing just under 10 000 hospital beds in the UK. The vast majority are in rural settings with around a quarter of them in Scotland. In Wales, apart from Aberystwyth, the North and South Wales coastal corridors and the Welsh valleys, the entire secondary care provision is by community hospital provision. Many community hospitals also have minor injuries units medically staffed by local GPs.

The definition of a community hospital is '*a hospital without resident medical staff where the first point of contact for medical services, whether routine or emergency, is through a local GP or GP practice*'.

GPs working in such hospitals do so under a variety of unsatisfactory pay arrangements with very defective terms of service and pay scales, none of which have been substantively reviewed since their inception in 1979, with the exception of minor adjustments in the early 1990s. Part of the April 2002 framework agreement on the new GP contract *Your Contract Your Future* was the commitment to look at reviewing pay and conditions for GPs working in community hospitals. Although such work is not part of General Medical Services, in almost all cases, such work is a practice activity and commitment. In many rural areas, the local populace expects involvement of the local GP practice in the staffing of the community hospital. Attempts by GPs working in such hospitals to improve their lot has in many cases been thwarted by the threat of closure of the hospital.

Key factors in settling the community hospital pay issues are:

- The GMS out-of-hours opt-out is a reality from January 2005. Most community hospitals currently are staffed as a marginal cost activity by GPs out of hours. From January 2005, this will become a complete lost opportunity cost and in the absence of a better deal many GPs might resign from their community hospital work.
- A well-run practice could find it much more profitable to concentrate their efforts on Enhanced Services provision in the practice and on scoring very highly in the Quality and Outcomes Framework than on devoting time to the community hospital.
- Community hospital work is not part of GMS; it is funded from the Hospitals and Community Health Services Treasury vote, not the GMS Treasury vote.
- Community hospital work is nothing whatsoever to do with GMS funding. No deal should be funded as an Enhanced Service. Community hospital work is not primary care.
- There is no legal compunction upon a GP to undertake community hospital work and the PCO has no right to attempt to bundle the offer of Enhanced Services for other primary care work conditional upon the practice undertaking the community hospital work.
- The European Working Time Directive (EWTD) comes into force in August 2004 for hospital doctors in training, thus highlighting to employers that it is already in force and should already apply to consultants and other specialist hospital grades. There are significant cost advantages to PCOs in contracting GP practices to undertake the work.
- It is of course possible, as it always has been, to dismiss the GPs, as they have no security of tenure. The PCO cannot be compelled to contract with GPs.

Rural isolated practices

Some practices operate in such isolation and to such small numbers of patients that doctors have to be induced to practise in such locations by means of a guaranteed net income and extra support for practice expenses. All but three inducement practices are located in Scotland and the arrangements in England, Wales and Northern Ireland will mirror the Scottish arrangements.

Under the new GMS contract, Inducement Practitioners (IPs) will have the choice of becoming salaried employees of the PCO, with contracts of employment based on the model contract described in the supporting documentation to *The New GMS Contract 2003: Investing in General Practice*. Alternatively, they may continue as independent practitioners, with their previous income and allowances protected by a specially designed MPIG arrangement, which recognises the specific payment arrangements for IPs. Arrangements for the continued employment of associates are also being negotiated. *See* Chapter 19 for further details.

Out-of-hours arrangements

The structures and skill mixes of staff utilised by the NHS to deliver out-of-hours services are beginning to change. No longer is the sole model one of out-of-hours provision by personal responsibility of service provision through GPs. Structures are evolving, utilising resources such as NHS Direct/NHS 24 as answering and preliminary triage of patients' problems. These services then hand the problem to any of a number of different agencies according to the nature of the problem presented. Greater use is to be made of the ambulance service and of paramedics, whose skill repertoire is increasing and at the minimum can be used to undertake basic physical examinations and to report the findings to a remotely located doctor for advice. From 1 January 2005 the PCOs become responsible for the provision of all out-of-hours care. There are no locations on the mainland of England, Wales and Northern Ireland which are too remote for PCOs to take responsibility for provision of out-of-hours services. In Scotland some of the remote islands and literally one or two mainland locations may prove impossible to cover other than by utilising the local general practitioners. Under such circumstances PCOs will have to put into place major and costly support structures to recompense the handful of GPs in question for the major differential impact such commitment places on their lives, and future recruitment issues will force PCOs to find a long-term solution.

Imaginative utilisation of healthcare facilities and community hospitals in rural areas will allow PCOs to take responsibility for the provision of out-of-hours care in a manner that a significant number of rural co-operatives have done, particularly since 1996.

Branch surgeries and extended service provision

For many years general practitioners practising in special geographical circumstances have had to provide an unresourced and unrewarded extended range of services at their surgeries. The most obvious examples are those of phlebotomy and near-patient testing. From April 2004 there is no obligation to provide such services unless they are specifically contracted for by the PCO as an Enhanced Service. Practitioners should not undertake such unresourced services in the future as not only will they not be paid for their efforts, but also there will be no means of recouping practice expenses which are incurred doing such work, which in future will be a simple act of charity.

Until April 2004 there has been discretion concerning the premises reimbursements for branch surgeries. In future if the premises are open 20 hours per week and staffed to provide a full range of Essential and Additional Services then the premises costs of such surgeries must be met by the PCO. This includes the costs of a real-time landline link for computers between the surgeries.

Immediate care and first responder services

A common feature of general practice in rural, remote or isolated areas is the ethical obligation to make a personal response by attending the scenes of medical and trauma emergencies. The provision of pre-hospital immediate care and first responder roles to victims of trauma and life-threatening illness is a service primarily fulfilled through the statutory ambulance services, usually by state-registered paramedics. In special geographical locations the ambulance service frequently cannot mount the traditional paramedic response to such incidents in less than 30–45 minutes and sometimes longer, even when a crew is available for tasking immediately. The local population by custom and practice will often phone the surgery in circumstances where in more populated or less remote areas they would have dialled 999. For social and professional reasons the GP has no option but to respond personally.

In certain geographical, operational, or clinical circumstances, an ambulance service or a paramedic may request the attendance, assistance and support of an appropriately trained general medical practitioner at the scene of a clinical emergency to provide clinical support and skills beyond those normally practised by general practitioners or paramedics.

Such work is currently unremunerated, and is very disruptive to the smooth running of a practice. The performance of such work requires the maintenance of extra skills and the use of additional equipment. In some parts of the UK PCOs have fully funded the training of GPs for such work and ambulance services have issued relevant equipment and supplies.

National specification and benchmarked pricing have been agreed as part of the new GMS contract for a National Enhanced Service for immediate care services. The purpose of the NES is to enable practices to augment the ambulance service paramedic at the request of the ambulance service in the management of cases (actual or expected). Full details of the NES are available in the supporting documentation to *The New GMS Contract 2003: Investing in General Practice.*

The performance of such work requires the maintenance of extra clinical and support skills and the use of additional equipment. In the modern practising environment it is necessary to maintain skills and competencies in a demonstrable manner.

Table 18.1: Value of the Immediate Care NES

Consumables purchased by	The practice	The PCO
Retainer	£1548	£1239
Fee per call in hours	£90	£60
Fee per call out of hours	£150	£120

Chapter 19

Scotland

Mary Church

Summary

- Scotland has a unique allocation formula.
- Choice of contractual arrangements for rural practices.
- Specific methodology for Inducement Practitioners.
- Choice of IM&T systems.
- Three year rolling programme of premises development.
- Enhanced out-of-hours payments for practices which cannot opt out.

Introduction

The new GMS contract in Scotland means GPs working in Scotland will be rewarded to reflect the distinctive circumstances and needs in Scotland relative to the rest of the UK. Devolution has resulted in unique health policies in Scotland which differ from the rest of the UK and are represented in the Scottish contract.

Scottish Allocation Formula (SAF)

Making use of a formula enables the distribution of the available resources among GP practices to reflect the relative needs of the Scottish practice population. The SAF does not inform the total size of the Scottish budget for the Global Sum. It is a population-based formula with a series of weightings to reflect:

- the age–sex structure of the practice population (demography)
- the additional need of the practice population (morbidity and deprivation)
- the rurality and remoteness of the practice population.

Other weights, applicable throughout the UK, reflect nursing and residential home patients, new registrations and a market forces factor for staff costs.

Derivation of Scottish weights

It is all very well being told how sensible using a Scottish formula is, without understanding the reasons for the differences. The age–sex consultation weights are based on data derived from Continuous Morbidity Recording (CMR) practices. Around 70 practices across Scotland provide the consultation information for this database.

To reflect accurately the socio-economic status of the Scottish population, an index of deprivation and mortality is included on the basis of the following indicators:

- the unemployment rate
- the proportion of elderly people claiming income support
- the standardised mortality rate amongst people under the age of 65
- households with two or more indicators of deprivation.

To recognise the additional costs needed to provide GMS in remote and rural areas, a further weighting is applied using the following indicators:

- the population density (hectares per resident)
- the population sparsity (the percentage of population living in settlements of less than 500 residents)
- the percentage of patients attracting road mileage payments.

The SAF will, therefore, allocate a Global Sum based on Scottish data and Scottish factors. It would be in no one's interest to destabilise practices simply due to the introduction of a new contract which brings with it new funding streams. To ensure this does not happen, the Scottish Executive will ensure that existing funding flows to practices for NHS Board Unified Budgets will continue.

Remote and rural arrangements

Securing help to areas with distinctive needs

The advantages of the new contract are not just for urban practices; rural communities can have all the benefits too. The excess costs in delivering GMS to remote and rural areas have customarily been borne by Scotland. Funds from fees and allowances were insufficient to maintain GMS services in rural areas and special arrangements had to be made to keep practices viable.

In order to ensure services for very sparsely populated communities in remote areas, 'essential' practices received support which provided a guaranteed level of income that was directly linked to the Intended Average Net Income (IANI). This focus on remote but essential practices is packaged as the Inducement Practitioner (IP) Scheme.

Even though this support is provided, working in a remote area requires a different time commitment. A variety of additional skills are needed in order to provide the range of services for patients not necessarily required of GPs working in less remote areas. The 24-hour out-of-hours obligation is probably the single most important disincentive to recruitment and retention, but GPs must also act as first responder, mental health officer, major incident office and provide minor injury and community hospital services. These responsibilities remain, needing proper reward and resourcing.

Inducement Practitioners (IPs)

Under the new contract IPs have the following options:

- independent contractor status with a Global Sum, Minimum Practice Income Guarantee (MPIG), quality payments, Enhanced Services payments and additional out-of-hours payment
- a salaried option
- the existing non-GMS contractual alternatives.

Calculating the GSE for IPs is done in two steps:

1   Add together:
    - the total value of the Global Sum Equivalent fees and allowances payments made to the practice in relation to the baseline year. This is the same set of fees and allowances that apply to all GMS practices and are as itemised in Annex D of the Statement of Financial Entitlements
    - the value of inducement payments made to the practice in relation to the baseline year.
2   From this figure, subtract the value of locum fees and expenses as claimed by the practice in relation to the baseline year.

For dispensing IPs an adjustment will be made to reflect the value of dispensing profit in relation to the baseline year.

The current level of entitlement will continue and the existing eligibility will remain unchanged.

Associates

The associate scheme will continue, although this is likely to be under different arrangements.

Out-of-hours services

The aim in Scotland is to ensure that the out-of-hours services keep running smoothly. In order to ensure stability and reliability, it is necessary to redesign an integrated service so that virtually all practices will be able to opt out of out-of-hours services.

A very few, extremely isolated practices may have to continue the provision of out-of-hours services but that does not mean development has finished. The new contract implementation group, the Scottish Executive and the SGPC will constantly strive to see what mechanisms can be put in place to achieve total opt-out. In the meantime the following special arrangements will apply:

- retention of the agreed out-of-hours abatement by the practice
- payment of the weighted capitation share of the Out-Of-Hours Development Fund and increased investment by the NHS Boards
- additional payment to cover any differential between the total of these and the locally determined payments to salaried GMS practitioners for providing out-of-hours cover
- other measures to support practices who cannot opt out will be provided by the PCO as described in the contract document *The New GMS Contract 2003: Investing in General Practice.*

IM&T

With GPASS, the Scottish Executive Health Department produced a publicly-funded clinical system, used by over 80% of Scottish practices. As with other UK-standard software, there are plenty of extra developments which will continue to be added to GPASS to meet the demands of the new contract. Scottish GPs will still have a choice of RFA-accredited GP clinical systems and those who continue or take up that option will be fully supported and will be tailored to fit with NHS Scotland's IM&T strategies. Specific guidance on Read codes is available from Scottish Clinical Information

Management in Primary Care (SCIMP) as part of the Clinical Effectiveness Programme website at www.ceppc.org/guidelines.

Premises

All premises funding will eventually be locally managed within the Board's Unified Budget. But, to meet existing commitments, transitional arrangements will ensure investment is targeted at the most appropriate localities and avoid exposure of third party landlords and developers to undue risk.

In the future, Boards will be expected to develop rolling three-year GP practice premises programmes. When agreement for funding from the centre has been reached, the revenue consequences should reassure GP practices their developments will be fully supported.

Cost rents, improvement grants and grants to surrender leases will continue to be met from NHS Boards' cash-limited Unified Budgets.

Branch surgeries

For isolated communities, branch surgeries offer vital access to health services. They could also act as centres for provision of a range of Enhanced Services. Therefore, closure decisions would need full consultation with the local population. Although they may be open for only a few hours a week, the essential nature of this provision will override virtually all other considerations in the need to keep a branch surgery open.

Dispute resolutions and appeals

When things are not running smoothly

Much as we would like it, contracts between two parties do not always run like a well-oiled machine. In order to maintain fairness, it is necessary to have dispute procedures that will sort out problems in a just and unprejudiced way.

In the first instance, the Board and the contractor must try to resolve the problem locally. In the event of a dispute, either party could invite the Area Medical Committee to participate in the discussions. This procedure does not apply to assignments to closed lists where it may not be practicable for the parties to attempt local resolution within a seven-day period between the determination of the assessment panel and the referral to Scottish Ministers.

In the event of the failure of local resolution, the matter can be referred to the Scottish Ministers, who will appoint a panel of three members as adjudicator. A much more streamlined system of dispute resolution has been introduced to avoid and minimise unnecessary delay. The adjudicator must ask within seven days of its appointment for any representations either party wishes to submit. Except in rare and unusual circumstances, this should be received within not less than two weeks, but not more than four weeks. The final decision will be given to the Scottish Ministers. For full details on the dispute procedure refer to Part 7 of the Scottish Regulations, paragraphs 82–85.

Chapter 20

Wales

Andrew Dearden

Summary

Main areas of difference between the Welsh version of the contract and that for other countries in the UK are:

- flexibilities and funding arrangements regarding premises developments
- the agreement of Wales-wide arrangements for some of the Directed and National Enhanced Services
- IM&T funding – continuing the Foundation Programme
- quality payments using Welsh disease prevalence data and Welsh average list sizes.

Introduction

In the main, all of the agreements contained within the new General Medical Services contract apply to the practices of Wales. Due to the nature of devolution, however, there are a few subtle differences. It is important to understand each difference and how it will apply to Welsh practices so that no misunderstandings will occur.

This chapter will highlight each difference within the new contract and explain its impact on GPs in Wales in an accompanying explanatory paragraph.

Investing in General Practice

We'll first look at the document *Investing in General Practice: The New General Medical Services Contract 2003*.

Premises flexibilities

Specific arrangements for implementation of the premises flexibilities and standards will be developed for Scotland, Wales and Northern Ireland. In Wales, separate allocation arrangements will apply to premises funding. From April 2004, subject to primary legislation, there will be a Welsh GMS Premises Fund that will be held by the National Assembly for Wales. Local Health Boards (LHBs) will be guaranteed baseline funding to support existing projects and projects that have already been agreed. Baselines will be uprated annually for property cost inflation. Decisions on growth money will be taken by the Assembly, taking account of the needs of LHBs as set out in their Estate Strategies and on specialist advice provided by Welsh Health Estates. (Paragraph 4.59 of *The New GMS Contact 2003: Investing in General Practice*.)

This is probably the most clear difference in the Welsh version of the contract. The plan as stated is for the premises money to be held at Assembly level. GPs, in collaboration with their LHBs, will have to apply to the Assembly for funding required in their Estate Strategies. The Assembly will then prioritise according to need.

Personal Medical Services

The planned total investment detailed in the document covers all practices including PMS practices. The English and Scottish Health Departments are considering the basis on which increases in PMS income will be calculated in future. At the time of writing, there are currently no PMS practices in Wales or Northern Ireland. (Paragraph 5.3.)

Service development

Under the new GMS contract there will be national arrangements to co-ordinate and facilitate the development of schemes designed to get the most out of the health services provided to patients. Part of this will be the development of alternative models of service provision within general practice. In Scotland, Wales and Northern Ireland existing arrangements will take forward this agenda. In England, there will be an integrated multidisciplinary group under the aegis of the Modernisation Agency working with relevant external bodies. (Paragraph 6.47.) In Wales, the Assembly, led by the Primary Care Division, will do this work.

GP performance

Unsatisfactory performance by an individual GP will be dealt with either through the monitoring, appraisal and revalidation arrangements to which all GPs will be subject or through the disqualification procedures presently set out in section 49 *et seq.* of the 1977 Act in England and Wales, sections 29 to 32E of the 1978 Act in Scotland, and Schedule 11 to the Health and Personal Social Services (NI) Order 1972. (Paragraph 7.32.)

This basically means that the current practice-based systems will remain the first step for most complaints. The patient has the right to complain directly to the LHB in the first instance or after an unsatisfactory outcome (in the patient's view) arising from the practice-based complaints system. If they are unhappy with the outcome of this second step, then they can appeal to the Assembly or the Health Ombudsman for Wales, as there are no Strategic Health Authorities in Wales similar to those in England.

GPs in Wales will be subject to the same legislation as the rest of the UK.

Performers' List

At present there is provision for three separate list arrangements for GPs: the Medical List for GP principals, the Supplementary List for non-principals and locums, and the complete Services List for PMS providers. Inclusion on one of these lists is a precondition of GPs performing primary medical care to patients. In England and Wales, these three lists will be merged into a single primary care performers' list. (Paragraph 7.33.)

Those on one of the three lists mentioned above will automatically be placed on the single list once it is established. Those joining the list for the first time (e.g. those who have just finished their vocational training schemes) will need to ensure that they have been included on the providers' list before they undertake any service provision as GPs. Those moving from other parts of the UK also have to ensure they have been accepted and included on the single providers' list for Wales before they are able to work in general practice in Wales. Employers will have a responsibility to ensure that anyone they employ to work for them is registered on the single providers' list for Wales.

The Supporting Documentation

In the Supporting Documentation (the second and larger of the two new contract documents, *The New GMS Contract 2003: Investing in General Practice*

– *Supporting Documentation*) there are more differences for Wales. Most of these are to do with the various Enhanced Services. Again, we will go through each one highlighting the Welsh aspect.

Directed Enhanced Service for access to General Medical Services

The Welsh target on access is: 'patients will be able to access an appropriate member of the primary care team within 24 hours of requesting an appointment and much sooner in an emergency'. There is recognition in the Assembly that this target will not be achieved immediately but will take some time. The Access Directed Enhanced Service, therefore, is due to continue through 2003–04, 2004–05 and 2005–06.

The target for access is characterised by the word 'appropriate'. This means just what it says, that the patient should have 'access to an appropriate member of the primary care team', not solely to the GP, as the target in England demands.

The agreement reached between the Assembly and GPC Wales is that every practice will receive a lump sum payment at the start of each year of £5000 (uplifted annually). The practice will have to apply via the standard Welsh application form.

There will be an additional 50 points paid under the quality framework for actual achievement of the target. The process by which achievement is to be confirmed is under discussion between the Assembly and GPC Wales.

Directed Enhanced Service for influenza immunisation for patients in the under-65s at-risk group

In the past, GPs in Wales have been paid for flu immunisations given to the over-65s at item of service rate B and to those in at-risk groups under 65 at item of service rate A. Although, at the time the documents were published, GPs in the rest of the UK were to be paid item of service rate B for under-65s in at-risk groups, we had not obtained the same for GPs in Wales. However, after further discussions with the Assembly on Enhanced Services in Wales, the item of service rate B payment for all immunisations of people under 65 years old in at-risk groups was agreed.

Quality Information Preparation Directed Enhanced Service

The agreement reached with the Assembly was that a payment of £2500 would be made per average practice in November 2003 and April 2004, dependent on the submission of the appropriate application form.

A further £800 per whole-time-equivalent GP under the Foundation Programme was also agreed. This extra money, specifically given to all GPs in Wales to aid them to work on summarising their notes and getting their electronic records into a form suitable for the Quality and Outcomes Framework, is not available to GPs in England in the same way.

National Enhanced Services for anti-coagulation monitoring and near-patient testing

It was agreed, after intensive discussions between the Assembly and GPC Wales, that there should be central funding in the first year (and each year thereafter the funds would be delegated to LHBs) for these two NESs. This means that both of these will be available to every GP in Wales. GPC Wales felt it vital that funds were made available to all GPs to pay them for work many had been doing for free in the past. The money was also kept at Assembly level until the LHBs had 'spent' it by giving it to GPs. The amount set aside in the Assembly's budget for these NESs is £100 per patient per year.

It has been left to LMCs and LHBs to meet locally and introduce these schemes where they have not previously been set up or to meet to discuss increasing the current payment in line with the money allocated for this service.

National Enhanced Service for patients suffering from drug misuse

As above, there was an agreement to fund this service for patients in Wales. £1 million was allocated for the first year. It was agreed that the payments for the service would exactly mirror the fees set out in the NES service outline. GPC Wales strongly advises GPs not to accept any contract to provide these services for payments less than the NES published levels.

IM&T

The following was detailed in a joint letter sent out by the Chairmen of the Assembly's Implementation Board and GPC Wales.

1 Maintenance Costs

Maintenance costs will be paid from 1 April 2003. Those practices, which have paid for maintenance costs incurred on or after 1 April 2003, will be able to claim refunds. Precise details of which items can be included will be contained within the Minimum IT Service Specification.

2 GP Clinical Information System Upgrades/New Installations

Those remaining practices, which have not yet joined the ICT Foundation Programme for General Medical Practices, will be funded 100% to do so. To qualify they must sign up to the aims and objectives of the Foundation Programme in their entirety (which includes system specifications, quality standards etc.).

Those practices that have signed contracts for GP clinical information system upgrades or new installations as part of the Foundation Programme on or after 1 April 2003 will be funded 100% to do so which will involve refunds if they have already paid any part of the 20% contribution which has previously been required.

The Welsh Assembly will fund this 20% additional contribution. LHBs will be required to initially fund this 20% contribution, which will be re-claimed via the existing financial mechanisms that support the Foundation Programme.

Quality payments

As disease prevalence will be factored into clinical quality payments on a country-specific basis, GPs in Wales will be paid according to Welsh prevalence data rather than using UK data. GPC Wales are in discussions with the Assembly on what exactly this will mean. It is likely that GPs in Wales will earn slightly less than GPs in England, with the same levels of disease prevalence, under the Quality and Outcomes Framework for providing the same level of quality, i.e. achieving the same number of points. This is due to GPs in Wales being judged on national disease prevalence in Wales, which is higher than the average for England as a whole.

However, GPC Wales negotiators have been given a reassurance by the Assembly that GPs in Wales will not be paid less overall under the new contract due to this political decision, imposed by the Government. Once details of the balancing arrangements are agreed with the Assembly, GPC Wales will inform all GPs and LMCs as soon as possible.

At the moment there is simply not the statistical information available to calculate exactly the financial effect of using Welsh data. This will be available once the quality practice-based disease prevalence data are available towards the end of 2004–05 year. Once these data are available, it will be possible to calculate the exact amount that the quality framework, using Welsh disease prevalence data, has underpaid GPs in Wales. Once this amount is agreed, we will work with the Assembly to make sure that this amount is paid to GPs in Wales and not used to fund investment in infrastructure or other parts of the NHS.

Chapter 21

Northern Ireland

Brian Dunn

Summary

- The new GMS contract negotiations heralded a new relationship, with Northern Ireland's direct involvement in the process.
- Separate negotiations were undertaken in Northern Ireland on the Directed Enhanced Services for access and Quality Information Preparation.
- Practices in Northern Ireland should be well placed to secure significant achievement in the Quality and Outcomes Framework.
- All practices should be able to opt out of providing out-of-hours services if they wish.
- IM&T modernisation is underway in Northern Ireland.

GPs in Northern Ireland have traditionally had similar terms of service to the rest of the UK. However, the Department of Health and Social Services and Public Safety in Northern Ireland is not bound to accept the recommendations of the Doctors' and Dentists' Review Body (DDRB) and Northern Ireland GPC is an autonomous committee and not a subcommittee of GPC like Scottish GPC and GPC Wales. Traditionally, the UK GPC negotiated terms of service for GB GPs and NIGPC and the Northern Ireland Department negotiated on the Northern Ireland implementation of these. Usually, there were few or minor changes made. NIGPC had no input into the evidence presented to the DDRB for GP remuneration and generally the Northern Ireland Department followed the recommendations, although recent initiatives such as PMS, the 'golden hellos' and 'golden handcuffs' were not introduced.

The new GMS contract marked a change in the relationship between NIGPC and the UK GPC. NIGPC was represented on the UK negotiating team for the first time. The DHSSPS was an observer to the negotiations between the GPC and the NHS Confederation and the contract was accepted both by NI GPs and the Minister for Health in the Northern Ireland Executive before the Assembly was suspended.

Northern Ireland has not suffered the recruitment and retention crisis experienced in the rest of the UK. It has, however, been evident that in recent years, the number of junior doctors applying for the GP training scheme has been decreasing and English PCTs have been targeting GP registrars and locums for recruitment. Traditionally, investment in primary care in NI has been lower than in Great Britain and if NI had been excluded from this substantial cash injection into primary care, there would have been an exodus of GPs to GB. A further gain for NI GPs is that, for the first time, the Technical Steering Committee, which has traditionally been a GB-focused body that advised the DDRB on GPs' earnings and expenses, will monitor primary care funding as part of the Northern Ireland Gross Investment Guarantee. This will protect the investment in primary care and will allow NI GPs to compare earnings directly with their colleagues in the other three countries.

Essential and Additional Services

It is unlikely that any practice in Northern Ireland will wish to avail themselves of the opportunity to opt out of Additional Services on the basis of workload pressure. Northern Ireland has not experienced the difficulties of other countries of the UK in recruiting principals and list sizes are lower than in England or Wales.

Enhanced Services

Northern Ireland has the longest hospital waiting lists in the UK. One of the aims of the new GMS contract was to resource and encourage the transfer of work from secondary care to primary care. Northern Ireland would then appear to be ideally placed to benefit from the contract. It is too early to judge whether the four Boards and DHSSPS will use the contract to reduce pressure on the secondary sector. Certainly the early indications are that they will not and that concerns about funding the Quality and Outcomes Framework may squeeze the budget for Enhanced Services and paradoxically GPs may be forced to return some work they are presently performing in primary care to the secondary sector, resulting in lengthening waiting lists.

Boards have a legal obligation to commission the six Directed Enhanced Services (DESs). GPs have preferred-provider status – i.e. are legally entitled to provide – three of them: access, Quality Information Preparation (QuIP) and childhood vaccinations and immunisations. The other three DESs – services to violent patients, minor surgery and influenza immunisations – must be commissioned but not necessarily from practices. However, at the time of transition, practices are best placed to provide these services. There are national agreements on the pay rates for childhood vaccinations and immunisations, influenza immunisation, minor surgery and services to violent patients. In Northern Ireland, access and QuIP have been negotiated as follows:

- *Access*: The practice will agree an access target with their Board. They have three years to work towards 48-hour access to a primary care professional. Exclusions to the target are appointments for non-GMS services (for instance, life insurance medicals, examination for solicitors' reports, form filling etc.), where the patient does not so request or in the course of treatment of a chronic illness. The primary care professional should be the most appropriate for the patient's condition and may be a GP, or a trust- or practice-employed nurse, podiatrist, physiotherapist etc. The practice will not be disadvantaged if a trust-employed primary care professional cannot meet the access target. If the practice achieves the access target, they will receive a second payment and can also claim 50 quality points. For 2003–04, the average practice (list size of 4917 patients) will receive £2500 in February 2004 on agreeing a target and £2500 in May 2004 on achieving it. In June 2004, they will receive £2580 on agreeing a target and a second payment of £2580 on achieving it in March 2005. In 2005–06, they will receive £5325, again in two instalments. Monitoring of the target has been agreed for the first year.
- *QuIP*: This has been agreed as a payment of £3500 per average practice in 2003–04 and should have been paid in February 2004. NIGPC has yet to agree the amount for 2004–05.

Quality and Outcomes Framework

Most practices in Northern Ireland will be well placed to achieve significant income from the quality framework. Practice computer systems are the same as in England and Wales, with EMIS, InPractice and TOREX being the major suppliers, along with Merlock, who market and support Healthysoft in NI. As requested by GPs, quality points will be weighted for prevalence. NI probably has higher prevalence in some disease areas (especially CHD) than England, and NI is probably disadvantaged by using NI-wide prevalence data rather than UK-wide data. This could mean GPs in Northern Ireland having to work harder to earn the same amount as a GP in England. To ensure consistency, national list sizes will be used. The average list size in Northern Ireland is 4917 whereas the average in England is 5891. It is likely that the smaller list size will compensate for the expected higher prevalence.

It is anticipated that the Central Services Agency responsible for GP payments will use QMAS (Quality Management and Analysis System), which is being developed in England, for payments under the quality framework. Full implementation will be dependent on the HPSS network linking all GP surgeries under the Health and Care Number project. This will enable practices to assess how they are performing and compare their progress with other practices in their Board area and in the rest of Northern Ireland. It will also allow Boards to assess how their practices are performing for financial management and planning.

Out of hours

The new GMS contract gives GPs the option to opt out of their out-of-hours responsibility from April 2004 and the right to opt out from 1 January 2005. It is not anticipated that any practice in Northern Ireland will be regarded as too remote to exercise this opt-out. Northern Ireland has a network of out-of-hours co-operatives and a commercial provider in Belfast. Contacts in the out-of-hours period tend to be higher in Northern Ireland than in GB (often double the number of contacts) and there is an absence of other supporting services such as NHS Direct, NHS 24 and walk-in centres. Most GPs will opt out and Boards are presently working on the alternative service. Whatever configuration this may take, GPs will continue to be involved, working for the new organisations. The number of GPs providing an out-of-hours service will decrease and other primary care professionals (e.g. nurses, social workers and pharmacists) will play a larger part in the delivery of out-of-hours services. It is hoped that new services will be in place by late summer/early autumn.

Information management & technology

Most practices in Northern Ireland have RFA99-compliant systems. This is partly due to the decision of DHSSPS not to support GPASS after 1999. This meant that those practices with GPASS systems (the majority in Northern Ireland) switched to other systems.

Several modernisation projects are presently being implemented. These, along with the new contract, will put NI GPs on a similar IM&T footing to the rest of the country. The Central Services Agency are presently installing the Exeter payment system that is used in England and Wales and this is being updated to deal with the new GMS contract.

The Health and Care Number project is beginning to roll out electronic links to all GPs in the Province. This will enable electronic registration links (an aid to 'clean' lists) and electronic laboratory links for all practices (essential for the quality framework). Electronic links will facilitate QMAS for data extraction of quality points for practice use (monitoring progress throughout the year), Central Services Agency use (practice payment and disease prevalence calculation) and Boards (monitoring progress of their practices throughout the year for financial monitoring and planning).

In Northern Ireland, the resources for IT modernisation have been passed to Boards and practices have had the opportunity to bid for minor upgrades and 100% reimbursement for maintenance.

Flexible working

Northern Ireland is different from the rest of the UK as there is not a problem in filling vacancies. Northern Ireland has around 1100 GPs and 150 vocationally trained GPs presently working as locums. Some of these locums are seeking posts as principals and others have been content to work sessions in general practice, sometimes combining these with hospital sessions. The new GMS contract will encourage flexibility in career options and it is likely that there will be an increase in salaried GPs, part-time working, an expansion of GPs with Special Interest, some GPs working exclusively for out-of-hours providers and others offering services to neighbouring practices and Boards under Enhanced Services.

Issues for DHSSPS and Boards

The new GMS contract is a UK contract. However, there are differences between the four countries that will inevitably lead to differences in implementation. The contract promised a Gross Investment Guarantee (GIG). This is really four GIGs – one for each country. Northern Ireland Boards do not have unified budgets and are therefore slightly more exposed to the risk of GP overperformance in the quality framework. This may lead to a conservative approach to defining the various elements of the Northern Ireland GIG, with less funding for Enhanced Services.

Boards will have the ability to commission or provide Additional and Enhanced Services. It is unlikely that many (if any) practices will not provide all the Additional Services. Boards will have a duty to provide the six Directed Enhanced Services. It is likely these will be offered to practices, but some Boards may seek to be imaginative. Boards may have to provide some of the DESs. Some GPs may decide not to provide the access DES, meaning that the Board will have to provide the access standard for patients of those practices.

Perhaps the biggest challenge for the Boards is the provision of an alternative out-of-hours service. It is likely that most (if not all) GPs will opt out of their 24-hour responsibility. Northern Ireland has little infrastructure for the provision of out-of-hours services in most areas, other than GP out-of-hours co-operatives. GPs will inevitably have a major part to play in whatever out-of-hours solution is proposed and the Boards recognise that if GPs are to retain an interest, they will expect a solution well in advance of the latest possible date of 31 December 2004. We have yet to see proposals for this, but it is likely there will be a uniform out-of-hours solution throughout Northern Ireland.

The future

The new GMS contract is the biggest change in general practice since 1948. Northern Ireland will benefit particularly from IM&T modernisation and the changes proposed under the Enhanced Services and Quality and Outcomes Framework. Will the contract invigorate General Medical Services? Only time will tell. It is interesting that the legislation presented to Parliament to underpin the new GMS contract enables DHSSPS to introduce PMS to Northern Ireland.

Information technology: the history and the vision

Brian Dunn

The development of IT systems in primary care

Information technology in general practice has grown in an unplanned and unsystematic manner. It has developed through a mixture of enthusiastic GPs and software companies identifying a niche in the market. GP computing started in the 1970s but it was not until VAMP and AAH Meditel started their 'free' computer schemes that IT took off in UK general practice. These schemes were funded by the computer companies selling anonymised data to fund the purchase and maintenance of the systems. GPs were encouraged to record all consultations and prescriptions issued and the companies developed multi-user GP systems where each GP had a terminal on their desk instead of one computer in the reception area. The VAMP scheme continues today as the General Practice Research Database (GPRD) and was one of the methods used to assess workload for the new GMS contract.

The countries of the UK also were different – especially Scotland, where the most used system continues to be GPASS, provided free of charge in Scotland and in Northern Ireland until 1999 by the Scottish Health Department. Elsewhere, the cost of GP IT purchase and maintenance was reimbursed by the Government under the Statement of Fees and Allowances, with 50% funding directly reimbursed and the remaining 50% coming in the indirect expenses element of GP income.

The 1990 contract boosted usage of IM&T systems in general practice with the need to search and produce reports for immunisation and cervical smear targets as well as providing systems for health promotion and chronic disease management. With the increased workload that was a product of the 1990 contract, many practices saw computerised repeat prescribing as one way of increasing efficiency and improving record keeping. Fundholding also encouraged computerisation with clinical systems and administrative systems receiving 75–100% reimbursement.

Fundholding saw the integration of clinical and administrative systems and while the success of the scheme still divides GPs, it did allow the development of IT systems to monitor referrals to secondary sector, monitor prescribing and assist in needs assessment of practice populations. Total purchasing pilots and primary care groups continued this commissioning/purchasing of care for populations supported by practice IT systems. The percentage of practices using computers has increased and presently only a small minority of practices are not computerised.

The development of GP systems was driven by enthusiasts and the computer suppliers responding to GPs' needs to fulfil their contractual requirements or, for some early enthusiasts, by research. There was little direct Government influence until electronic registration of patients and item-of-service claims led to Health Authorities establishing electronic links with practices. This led to a desire from Government for standardisation of systems and eventually the development of Requirements for Accreditation (RFA) and NHSnet. The new GMS contract, however, heralds a change where Government both centrally and locally via PCOs will drive the IM&T agenda.

An integrated IM&T service

The development of computer processors and data storage has been exponential. Ten years ago, practices had computer systems with 40 megabyte hard disks – now disks are 40 to 80 gigabytes, i.e. one to two thousand times more storage. Other methods of data storage – CD and DVD – are commonplace and information is routinely transmitted electronically both at home and at work.

GPs initially connected their practice computers for electronic patient registration and item-of-service links. With the advent of NHS intranets, much more use can be made of links with PCOs, providers and sources of clinical information. The new NHS number in England and Wales (and its equivalent in Scotland and Northern Ireland) enables unique identifiers to be used to identify patients electronically for:

- registration – this helps to 'clean' lists
- communication – with PCO and secondary/community sector
- payment – for the Quality and Outcomes Framework

- PCO financial planning – anonymised data allowing PCOs to monitor global quality points achievement throughout the financial year
- needs assessment for PCOs and central government
- giving out-of-hours organisations access to practice medical records in the treatment of patients
- A&E access to GP records to assist in the treatment of patients
- electronic prescribing.

An integrated IM&T service means that GPs and the clinical system suppliers will no longer be the main drivers in the development of IT systems for use in general practice. Integration means that while the systems will be used by GPs and their staff, the GP system is one component of a NHS-wide system. Some of these systems may have a large central server with the data shared within the PCO and confidentiality enshrined for the consultation between GP and patient.

Integration fits into the Government's Integrated Care Records Service (ICRS) project and the present GP clinical system suppliers will have to provide compliant systems or the end may be in sight for independent suppliers. We have already seen some PCOs imposing IT solutions on GP practices. This contract guarantees GPs a choice of clinical system and there is no reason to impose a central solution on all practices as practices are different and have varying organisations and working methods.

Integrated Care Records Service (ICRS)

ICRS developed from the Wanless Report and the National Programme for IT (NPfIT). Wanless proposed doubling the amount spent on NHS IT, national data standards and central management of IT. NPfIT has four objectives:

- the development of robust IT infrastructure
- an electronic prescriptions service
- electronic bookings of appointments
- a life-long NHS health record service.

ICRS is the Government's vision for the life-long health record service. It is a centrally driven policy with, so far, little input from clinicians. The programme has a huge budget but many feel its aims are unachievable. The programme envisages Local Service Providers (LSPs) procuring and providing systems and all data captured (without clinician or patient consent) held on the 'NHS Spine' – a central database accessible to all within the NHS. Data are initially held in encrypted form and the patient must give consent for all data to be made available for perusal throughout the NHS. The programme raises many issues for doctors:

- confidentiality
- data quality
- interpretation of data recorded in one discipline by another
- GMC and data protection issues
- conflict with the RCGP/GPC guidance on paperless practices.

It is not possible to deal in detail with ICRS in this book, but an awareness of Government policy may help GPs interpret policy decisions by PCOs in implementing the IT aspects of the new GMS contract. The concept of LSPs is specified in the IT guidance for the contract, and implementation of NPfIT objectives appears to be embedded in the infrastructure being developed.

Bibliography

The documents below are either English or UK publications. The legislation can be found at www.legislation.hmso.gov.uk, the joint documentation between the BMA and the NHS Confederation can be found at www.bma. org.uk/gpcontract, and the Department of Health documentation can be found at www.dh.gov.uk/policyandguidance/humanresourcesandtraining/ modernisingpay/gpcontracts/. Where they are English, equivalent versions will exist for the other three countries. Readers should refer to the Health Departments' own websites for details of the equivalent legislation and documentation.

Primary legislation

- *Health and Social Care (Community Health and Standards) Act 2003.*

Secondary legislation

- *NHS (GMS Contracts) Regulations* (SI 2004/0291).
- *GMS Transitional and Consequential Provisions Order* (SI 2004/0433).
- *NHS (Performers Lists) Regulations* (SI 2004/0585).
- *Primary Medical Services (Directed Enhanced Services) (England) Directions.*
- *NHS (General Medical Services – Premises Costs) (England) Directions.*
- *GMS Statement of Financial Entitlements 2004–05 Directions.*

Contract documentation

- BMA General Practitioners Committee and NHS Confederation (March 2003) *The New GMS Contract 2003: Investing in General Practice.*
- BMA General Practitioners Committee and NHS Confederation (May 2003) *The New GMS Contract 2003: Investing in General Practice – Supporting Documentation.*
- Chisholm J and Farrar M (17 April 2003) *New GMS Contract – Joint Letter to all GPs.* BMA General Practitioners Committee and NHS Confederation.

- Chisholm J and Farrar M (30 May 2003) *New GP Contract: Latest Developments and Ballot – Joint Letter to all GPs.* BMA General Practitioners Committee and NHS Confederation.
- Department of Health (December 2003) *Delivering Investment in General Practice: Implementing the New GMS Contract.*
- Department of Health (March 2004) *Standard GMS Contract.*
- Department of Health (March 2004) *Default Contract.*

Index